The Best Mediterranean Diet for Healthy Weight Loss

30 Day Guide with 90 Easy to Cook Recipes

Introduction

I want to thank you and congratulate you for downloading the book, *"A Beginner's Mediterranean Diet for Healthy Weight Loss"*.

Why a Mediterranean Diet?

According to the **Mayo Clinic**, *"Research has shown that the traditional Mediterranean Diet reduces the risk of heart disease."* The Mayo Clinic went on to state "The Mediterranean diet is also associated with a **reduced incidence of cancer, and Parkinson's and Alzheimer's diseases**. Women who eat a Mediterranean diet supplemented with extra-virgin olive oil and mixed nuts may have a reduced risk of breast cancer."

In a recent **WebMD** article named **"The MIND Diet May Help Prevent Alzheimer's"**, it states that "Researchers have found that **people who stuck to a diet that included foods like berries, leafy greens, and fish had a major drop in their risk for the memory-sapping disorder, which affects more than 5 million Americans over age 65.**"

This book has the latest research about the Mediterranean Diet:

- Its benefits and the science behind it

- Authentic, easy to follow recipes

- A 30-day healthy, pragmatic lifestyle approach.

- Each chapter provides "author's tips" and Internet resources for additional help.

The people living in around the Mediterranean area are some of the healthiest in the world. Therefore, it is safe to say that the Mediterranean diet is one of the healthiest diets in the world. ***What makes it so special is its ability to bring about effortless weight loss and to fight chronic diseases like diabetes, Alzheimer's, heart disease, hypertension, stroke and many others***.

So, what comes to your mind at the thought of the term 'Mediterranean diet'? For many people, the mention of Mediterranean diet triggers thoughts of pasta and pizza from Italy, or lamb chops from Greece. But the truth is, that's not all there is to Mediterranean diet.

In fact, a true Mediterranean diet mainly comprises of seafood, fruits and veggies, hearty grains, olive oil and various other foods, which can greatly help you to fight against all manner of diseases and bring about good health. And the good news is that the diet also helps you follow a lifestyle that improves your general heath. Most of all, it is delicious too.

So, if you are looking to lose weight and acquire a clean bill of health in the process then the Mediterranean diet is the diet for you.

By reading this guide, you are going to learn what the diet is, the benefits that come with following the diet, how you can start following it and incorporate it into your lifestyle and the tips and strategies that you can use to increase your success rate in the diet.

This book is also going to provide you with **recipes that you can follow for up to 30 days** to help ease your transition from the conventional diet that you are in into the Mediterranean diet.

Get started now to systematically transform your life to reach your long-term lifestyle goals for permanent and healthy weight loss.

Thanks again for downloading this book and I hope you enjoy it!

The information herein is offered for informational purposes solely, and is universal as so. The presentation of the information is without contract or any type of guarantee assurance.

DISCLAIMER: *Everyone, regardless of their condition, should first consult with their physician or medical professional and receive formal medical clearance before starting any diet, lifestyle change or exercise program.*

This publisher and author are not licensed or medical practitioners and do not provide any medical advice whatsoever. The publisher and author claim no responsibility to anyone or entity for any liability, loss, or damage caused or allegedly caused by use of the information presented in this publication.

The trademarks that are used are without any consent, and the publication of the trademark is without permission or backing by the trademark owner. All trademarks and brands within this book are for clarifying purposes only and are the owned by the owners themselves, not affiliated with this document.

Table of Contents

Mediterranean Diet: A Comprehensive Background
What Is It?

When you think about the Mediterranean ways of life, a couple of things usually come to mind one, of them being how the Mediterranean people love eating foods like hummus, pizza, pasta and gyros. So, is that the Mediterranean diet? The answer is no. The diet is actually quite the opposite. So then, what exactly is a Mediterranean diet?

Contrary to popular belief, a Mediterranean Diet is not a diet per se but a pattern of eating that is popularly known for weight loss, prevention of multiple diseases and overall health improvement.

The diet was originally founded on the traditional eating habits of people in countries surrounding the Mediterranean Sea in the 1940's and 1950's. Some of these countries included Greece, Spain and Italy.

The diet basically emphasizes on the consumption of natural unprocessed whole foods. When you are on the diet, the general rule is for you to eat large amounts of vegetables, fruits, whole grains, healthy fats, sea foods, legumes like beans and olive oil. This is because these are the foods that made up the traditional meals that kept the Mediterranean people exceptionally healthy as compared to the people living in the U.K and the U.S back in the days.

While the Mediterranean Diet is more of a lifestyle than a diet, the question you might be having is:

Is There a Right Way of Following This Diet?

A lot of diets out there normally have an exclusive formula that you are usually required to follow in order to achieve success in those diets. When it comes to the Mediterranean diet, things are usually a bit different. There is no one right way of doing the diet. Let me break it down for you.

As you saw earlier, people from countries around the Mediterranean Sea were generally very healthy. That said, those people didn't eat the same exact things.

This is because the Mediterranean Sea is surrounded by different countries which have different cultures and are exposed to different types of foods. For instance, countries that are near the sea mostly ate sea foods while those that are far from the sea ate chicken and beef.

But they were all exceptionally healthy despite eating not so similar types of foods. This shows that there is no one strict way of following this diet and that the foods advocated in the diet are just a general guideline of foods to consume and not a food list that is written on stone. And that's one of the beauties of this diet. It gives you the freedom to adjust the foods provided in the diet to fit your needs and preferences.

That said, there are some general principles of the Mediterranean diet that we all need to follow if we are to replicate the level of health success and leanness that the people around the Mediterranean Sea enjoyed.

Here are the general principles:

- While on the diet, you should mostly focus on eating plant based foods such as nuts, legumes, whole grains, fruits and vegetables.

- You should stop or minimize the use of salt and instead use herbs and spices to flavor your food.

- You should try and consume poultry or fish at least twice in a week.

- You should limit your intake of red meat to at least a few times in a month.

- If you are to drink wine, which the diet allows you to do, you should keep your consumption to a minimum.

- You should stop using butter in cooking food and instead opt for healthy fats like canola oil and olive oil. If you have to use butter, ensure to limit how much butter you use.

- You should try and get plenty of exercise since people around the Mediterranean Sea were very active people.

Why Are the General Principles So Important?

They are important because people back then used to live a rural lifestyle where they only ate what they grew and caught from the sea, which is totally opposite of how we eat and live today.

Today, we not only eat farm harvested foods but also manufactured and processed foods, which are full of unhealthy chemicals and additives. So, the general principles normally just help you stay on course by highlighting what you should not compromise even as you enjoy the freedom to choose what you want to eat.

How Easy Is It to Follow the Mediterranean Diet?

Have you ever been on a diet that made you starve yourself in order to be lean? I know this has never been the case, right? Did you at least smile with my crazy comment?

Well, thankfully the Mediterranean diet is not one of those diets. This diet usually goes easy on you when it comes to rules. It does not impose unrealistic and unbearable rules to you like most of the diets do.

Here are four points that will show you just how easy the diet is:

• *The Mediterranean Diet does not require you to starve yourself:* In fact, it usually encourages you to eat 3-5 times in a day so long as you eat small portions of foods or you eat what you need to fill satisfied and not what you need to feel excessively full.

This makes the diet very easy to follow and adopt as a lifestyle because it enhances what comes natural to you which is eating when you are hungry.

> • *It reduces your hunger:* The Mediterranean diet typically contains foods that are rich in fiber and healthy fats, which usually fills you up for long periods of time. This normally eliminates the frequent hunger that makes other diets unbearable.

- *In a Mediterranean diet, no one tells you to count your calories or what food groups to avoid completely:* You have the control.

Here, you are given the freedom to figure out how many calories you want to take to lose weight. This is after you have been guided on what to consume and how to consume it in order to lose weight (this will be explained further in the subsequent chapters).

In addition to that, the diet does not ban entire food groups like most weight loss diets do. The only advice to you is what to avoid from the different food groups, which still enables you to have something to eat from each food group.

- *The diet allows you to have a glass of wine or two in a day:* I like this! One of the amazing things about the Mediterranean diet is how it allows you to have a glass of wine. I mean, who doesn't like a glass of wine after a hard-working day or after a tantalizing meal.

So, as you can see, the Mediterranean Diet is pretty easy to adopt and follow because it does not restrict and pin you down to very strict. We both know that unnatural or very restrictive eating habit are not sustainable long-term.

That said, you can't help but wonder why you should follow the Mediterranean Diet? What makes it so special?

The chapter below is going to answer that by highlighting for you the health benefits that make the Mediterranean Diet a must follow diet.

Benefits of a Mediterranean Diet

The Mediterranean Diet is regarded as one of the healthiest diets in the world and that is because it has been discovered to boost human health, help in weight loss, and help in the prevention of various diseases.

In this chapter, you are going to learn the health benefits that make a Mediterranean Diet a worthwhile diet to follow.

Below is a list of 5 extensively explained benefits that you stand to gain when on a Mediterranean Diet:

1. *It helps you lose weight*

One of the key benefits of a Mediterranean Diet is how it helps you lose weight.

So how does it do that? When you adopt a Mediterranean diet, there are three small lifestyle changes that the diet usually makes you make.

- First, it makes you lower the portion size of your meals. This is usually a very important change because one of the reasons why you gain weight is because of overeating.

  When you overeat, you normally end up with a surplus of energy in your body which only ends up being stored as fat. That process is what makes you gain weight.

The Mediterranean Diet normally puts a stop to that process of weight gain by making you eat small portions of meals that only supply your body with the energy that it needs and nothing more. I know you are thinking; won't this make you hungrier and lead to unnecessary snacking?

The answer is no. The Mediterranean Diet contains foods that are rich in fiber which means they fill you up more and eliminate the frequent feeling of hunger. This makes you snack less and eat less during your meals. Less consumption of unnecessary food leads to less fat accumulation and a stop to weight gain.

• Secondly, the diet makes you focus on healthy fats like monounsaturated fats and polyunsaturated omega 3 fatty acids. When you consume large portions of those fats, your body becomes more accustomed to burning fat for energy as opposed to using glucose for energy because the diet is usually very low in glucose.

The burning of fat for energy normally enables your body to reduce your stored body fats by constantly burning them for energy. That helps you lose weight in an immense way.

• Thirdly, the diet advise that you exercise regularly. The process of exercising usually raises your body's energy demand. This automatically does two things in your body.

For starters, it makes you use up all the glucose in your system, which avoids the storage of surplus glucose that leads to weight gain. Secondly, it makes your body to start burning fats for energy in order to meet the body's rising energy demand. This helps you lose weight.

The combination of the above three points are the reason why a Mediterranean Diet is known for fast weight loss.

2. *It improves the health of your heart*

The other benefit that you stand to gain from following a Mediterranean Diet is the improvement of your heart's health. A lot of us today have a bad bill of health when it comes to our hearts. This is mostly because we consume foods which make us more prone to heart related illnesses like bad fats and avoiding regular exercise.

The Mediterranean Diet usually improves your heart health by discouraging the consumption of bad fats like hydrogenated oils (Trans fats) and saturated fats. These fats promote higher LDL (low-density lipoprotein)/bad cholesterol that builds up deposits in your arteries, which could then cause heart attacks.

Instead of bad fats, the diet encourages you to consume heart healthy fats like polyunsaturated and monounsaturated fats like olive oil, canola oil and nuts. These fats usually contain a type of Omega 3 fatty acid called linolenic acid, which helps in lowering blood clotting and decreasing the level of triglycerides in your body (the two are associated with sudden heart attacks).

The acid also helps in moderating your blood pressure and improving your blood vessels which are all efforts that help in reducing the level of LDL cholesterol in your body and promoting the level of HDL (High-density lipoproteins)/good cholesterol that improves the health of your heart.

3. *It Prevents Cancer*

There was a large study that was carried out and published in the International Journal of Cancer. This study concentrated on the lives of over 62,000 women who followed the Mediterranean Diet to see how that affected their risk of breast cancer over a period of 20 years. The study eventually discovered that those women who followed the Mediterranean Diet exclusively had a 40% reduced risk of getting breast cancer.

This can be translated to mean that the Mediterranean diet is also good at potentially preventing cancer. But how does it do it?

Well, it does this by providing you with a nutrition that promotes the reduction of inflammation in your body and oxidative damage.

Inflammation is part of our body's immune system, which helps us fight any external enemies like bacteria and chemical irritants that can hurt our health. That said, inflammation has a dark side where it can overstay its welcome when it travels to your cells to fight bacteria.

The dark side of inflammation has been seen to promote growth of tumor, which causes cancer. Oxidative damage is one of the factors that usually increase the inflammatory response, which as you saw above leads to the development of cancer.

The Mediterranean Diet protects you from cancer by providing you with a diet that is abundant in antioxidant rich vegetables and fruits, which increase the total antioxidant capacity in your body that reduce oxidative load and oxidative damages. By reducing oxidative damages, it automatically reduces the inflammation in your body; a powerful tool in the formation of cancer.

4. It Controls Your Blood Pressure

A study that was published in the European Journal of Clinical Nutrition Vol. 63 established that Mediterranean style of eating that is rich in olive oil, vegetables and fruits can reduce the risk of high blood pressure or hypertension.

How does it do that?

First of all, the risk of high blood pressure is normally increased by the presence of high sodium content in your blood. Well, for starters, the fruits and vegetables on the Mediterranean Diet are usually low in sodium content. So, when you consume them, you create an environment that decreases your risk of high blood pressure.

Secondly, the vegetables, fruits and olive oil that you usually consume from a Mediterranean diet normally contain potassium, which is a mineral that maintains proper heart functions, which improves blood flow which in turn reduces your risk of getting high blood pressure.

Thirdly, and most importantly, the combination of unsaturated fatty acids and nitrogen that come from the consumption of olive oil and vegetables usually form a fatty acid known as 'nitro' fatty acids. This fatty acid usually blocks the enzyme sEH (soluble epoxide hydrolase) responsible for raising blood pressure.

The combination of the three facts above is what makes a Mediterranean Diet so good at preventing or reducing the occurrence of high blood pressure.

5. It Improves the Quality of Your Skin

One of the most sought-after procedures in the universe today are surgeries meant to improve the skin and reduce the signs of an aging skin. This might surprise you but one of the natural ways of improving the quality of your skin and reducing the aging signs from it is actually by following a healthy diet like the Mediterranean Diet.

The Mediterranean diet usually gets rid of what affects your skin negatively. So, what affects your skin negatively?

The answer is refined carbohydrates and processed foods. These types of foods normally contain a lot of sugar, which promote inflammation that leads to the breakdown of collagen, a fibrous protein that makes your skin firm.

The Mediterranean Diet prohibits the use of the above food types and that automatically puts a stop to the rate at which your skin forms wrinkles and sags after collagen is broken down.

However, that is not all that the Mediterranean Diet does to improve the quality of your skin. It also provides you with vegetables, olive oils, fatty fish and nuts which are rich in antioxidants that your body uses to repair skin damage. The foods also contain healthy fats that increase the elasticity of your skin. Therefore, adopting a Mediterranean Diet can slow the aging process of your skin and make you have a young and vibrant looking skin.

These are not the only benefits that you can get by following a Mediterranean Diet. With the diet, you can also expect to have an easier time when fighting diabetes, reducing your risk of suffering from Parkinson's disease as well as Alzheimer's disease and much, much more.

That said, following a Mediterranean Diet and enjoying the above benefits is usually not an easy task especially for beginners like you. This is because there is a lot of information out there about the diet that most often than not mislead beginners and make them follow the wrong instructions which leads them to failure.

The next chapter is going to debunk some of the myths that you are likely to get out there when you start following the diet. Check it out below.

Mediterranean Diet Myths Debunked

As you saw above, following a Mediterranean diet has a lot of benefits. However, not many people get to enjoy those benefits. This is because there is a lot of information out there that either discourages them from following the diet or misleads them and makes many people to do the wrong things while on the diet. Some of these myths normally affect beginners like you because you do not know a lot about the diet so it's easy for you to fall for any piece of information.

However, this should not worry you. This guide has got your back and will help you dodge that bullet of failure by highlighting for you the common myths and misconceptions that you are likely to come across in your journey to weight loss.

Myth 1: The Mediterranean Diet Is Very Expensive

As a beginner, you are likely to come across information that a Mediterranean Diet is too expensive to follow. This is a big misconception that has been spreading around for years now. Yes, a Mediterranean diet can be quite expensive but there are ways that you can use to make the diet fit your budget or become pocket friendly.

- For starters, you can buy your foods/ingredients in bulk. Buying in bulk is usually cheaper than buying small portions of foods.

- Secondly, you can buy your foods at the farmer's market when it's about to be closed. Foods from the farmers market are usually less expensive but you can get them even cheaper if you go to the market later in the day. Farmers and growers hate packing their produce back up so they usually reduce their price when they are about to close.

• Thirdly, you can eat more of vegetables and less of meat, which will save you a lot of cash and make your meals cheaper and affordable. I realize this may be difficult for some of you but maybe you can reduce the amount of meat over time.

• The fourth way you can use is to adopt a behavior of buying products when they are on discount and then freeze them for later use.

The Mediterranean Diet is pretty affordable and easy to adopt irrespective of your level of income.

Myth 2: You Can Eat All the Cheese That You Want When on a Mediterranean Diet

This is a huge misconception. Incorporating cheese in your meals and eating it is a common practice in the Mediterranean Diet. However, cheese is only supposed to be consumed in moderation. If you eat a lot of cheese then you will consume unwanted calories which will end up making you gain weight.

Myth 3: You Can Drink as Much Wine as You Want

This is another huge misconception that has been going around you may have heard. Wines normally have some unique health benefits for your heart. But that is only true when you drink it in moderation which can be one or two glasses a day. If you drink more than that, then the wine can become unhealthy to your heart and can also slow down your weight loss progress due to sugars and carbohydrates in the wine.

Myth 4: The Mediterranean Diet Is About Eating Huge Meals

One of the most popular myths about Mediterranean diet is that you can eat huge meals like people around the Mediterranean Sea and you will still lose weight. This is a huge misconception.

People around the Mediterranean Sea do not lose weight and stay lean by eating huge meals but by eating small servings of low calorie Mediterranean food. Huge meals normally accumulate into high calorie intake which can easily spill over into excess energy that your body stores as fat.

As a beginner therefore, you should never pay follow this myth, as it can affect your weight loss progress.

Myth 5: You Don't Have to Exercise When You Are on the Mediterranean Diet

This myth is partly true although the mindset behind it is misleading and untrue. The Mediterranean people who enjoyed a lot of success with this lifestyle diet 50 to 60 years ago never went to the gym to exercise.

This means you don't necessarily need to go to the gym to succeed in this diet. That part I agree with the people that spread this myth.

The part that you shouldn't fall for because it is untrue and misleading is the part of this myth that implies you do not need to exercise or become physically active when on a Mediterranean Diet if you are not already.

The Mediterranean people never needed to exercise because their daily lives were full of physically challenging activities. For example, they did a lot of manual work because they had no access to machines.

They also walked a lot to get to where they were going since there weren't as too many cars back then as there is today. That was their exercise.

Today, we have the privilege of not doing manual labor and walking for long distances because we have machines that have taken over manual labor and cars that are readily available to take us where we want. This means for us to replicate the physical activity that the Mediterranean people did, we need to do some form of exercise regularly. This means you need to exercise when on a Mediterranean diet.

Myth 6: Eating Large Portions of Pasta and Bread Is Allowed

As a beginner, many people will tell you that eating large portions of pasta and bread is the Mediterranean way of life. And isn't that what many Mediterranean's eat especially the Italians? The answer is yes and no.

Italians eat a lot of pasta with bread but what you might not know is that they eat very small portions of those foods. In fact, pasta is usually a side dish to them. They eat it with vegetables, salads, bread and meat.

In short, how they eat pasta and bread does not affect their chances of losing weight on the diet and succeeding in it because they do it in moderation.

Therefore, as a beginner you should never eat large portions of pasta and bread as it will interfere with your weight loss progress. What you should do is eat small portions of pasta and bread. Over time, you may be able to moderate the exact amount that work for you the best.

Now that you are aware of the misleading myths, the next step is for you to learn how to start following the Mediterranean Diet.

Check this out in the chapter below.

How to Start Following the Mediterranean Diet

All the above chapters have been leading to this very chapter, which is how you can get started into the Mediterranean diet as a beginner. As you saw above, a Mediterranean Diet is an easy to follow diet. In fact, some people refer to it as a common-sense approach of eating and living. The simplicity of it makes it easier to follow.

This chapter is going to explain to you the easy process that you need to follow in order to start following the Mediterranean Diet. This process will be highlighted in step form.

Let's get down to it starting with the first step below.

Step 1: Know What to Eat and What Not to Eat

For you to follow a Mediterranean Diet, you need to first know what you are allowed to eat and what you are not allowed to eat on the diet. Below is a list of the guidelines of what you can eat, what you are allowed to eat in moderation and what you are not allowed to eat.

What to Eat on the Mediterranean Diet

Here are the foods that you are encouraged to eat when you start following a Mediterranean Diet.

Vegetables and fruits

The main foods that you are recommended to consume when you are on a Mediterranean Diet are vegetables and fruits. Good examples of vegetables and fruits to consume include carrots, cauliflower, eggplant, artichoke, onions, spinach, kale, broccoli, tomatoes, olives, apples, grapes, strawberries, oranges and bananas.

Whole grain and potatoes

Whole grains and potatoes are the other important type of foods that you need to consume when on a Mediterranean diet. Some good sources of whole grain foods and potatoes include whole oats, buckwheat, couscous, barley, rye, brown rice, whole wheat pasta, whole wheat bread, sweet potatoes, turnips and white potatoes.

Seafood

Seafood like fresh fish are good sources of proteins. Other seafood that you can eat include crabs, mussels, oysters, lobsters, shrimp, tuna, haddock and salmon. Stay with the wild-caught fish and not the farm-raised variety which are raised in waters that may be polluted and fed with antibiotics along with artificial coloring with salmon.

Healthy fats

Healthy fats are a major part of the Mediterranean Diet. This is because they provide you with an alternative meal when you get rid of unhealthy fats like butter (although I admit that I love butter). Good sources of healthy fats when used in moderation include coconut oil, avocado oil, extra virgin oils avocados and olives.

Nuts and seeds

Nuts and seeds are good sources of healthy fats and proteins. Some of them include pumpkin seeds, sunflower seeds, cashews, hazelnuts, walnuts and walnuts. While nuts are good for you, just beware that nuts contain a lot of calories so they should be enjoyed in moderation.

Legumes

Good sources of legumes include chickpeas, peanuts, lentils, peas and beans. Be careful with peanuts as allergies from eating them seem to be more common.

Herbs and spices

Some of the great spices and herbs include mint, rosemary, cinnamon, basil and pepper. Cinnamon is great because it is high in antioxidants. Be sure to use the Ceylon version of cinnamon if you decide to take it regularly.

Water

Water usually helps you to hydrate your body, which is very important when it comes to weight loss. It also makes you feel full but it is good for you overall. After all, your body is about 70% water.

What You Are Allowed to Consume in Moderation

Below is a list of foods that you should only eat occasionally. This is because they are unhealthy if you eat them frequently.

- Red meat; they include bacon, ground beef and steak. If I eat red meat, I choose to only eat grass fed beef rather than corn fed beef which has a much higher level of Omega 6 oils.

- Dairy; it includes low fat milk, cheese and yogurt. Low fat and fat free dairy is acceptable.

- Eggs; a good source for protein

- Poultry; they include duck, turkey and chicken.

- Wine. I prefer red but white is fine as well.

What You Are Not Supposed to Eat

Below is a list of foods that you need to stay away from when you are on a Mediterranean Diet.

- Processed meat; good examples are sausages and hot dogs. These are generally not good for you regardless. However, you can easily find bacon and hot dogs cured naturally and without the harmful nitrates.

- Refined oils; good examples of these include cottonseed oil, vegetable- oil and soybean oil.

- Added sugars; like sodas, chocolate, sweets, candy and ice creams. Hidden sugars can be found in food products such as ketchup, spaghetti sauce and many others. Read the ingredient labels closely.

Latest research has also shown that diet sodas can be very bad for you as well due the artificial ingredients and possibly making your body crave sugar to the low-calorie sweeteners fooling your body.

- Saturated or trans fats; like butter and margarine. My vote that if you use butter occasionally and in moderation, you should be fine.

- Processed foods; many foods that come in packages have unhealthy fats and preservatives to keep the food from getting rancid to extend their shelf life in the stores.

Step 2: Learn the Dietary Guidelines for a Healthy Balanced Diet

The second step after learning what you can and can't eat in a Mediterranean Diet is for you to learn the composition and servings of those foods you need to eat on a daily and monthly basis. For you to know that, you need to understand the Mediterranean diet pyramid.

The Mediterranean diet pyramid is a guide that shows you what you need to eat frequently, moderately and what portions of those foods are good for optimum health and weight loss. Below is a picture of the Mediterranean diet pyramid.

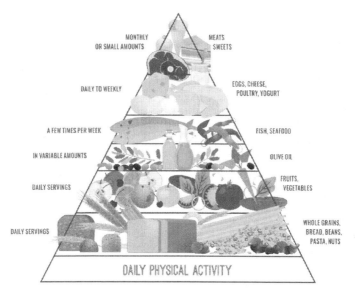

MONTHLY OR SMALL AMOUNTS — MEATS SWEETS

DAILY TO WEEKLY — EGGS, CHEESE, POULTRY, YOGURT

A FEW TIMES PER WEEK — FISH, SEAFOOD

IN VARIABLE AMOUNTS — OLIVE OIL

DAILY SERVINGS — FRUITS, VEGETABLES

DAILY SERVINGS — WHOLE GRAINS, BREAD, BEANS, PASTA, NUTS

DAILY PHYSICAL ACTIVITY

MEDITERRANEAN DIET

As you can see, the Mediterranean Diet pyramid is normally broken down into daily, weekly and monthly foods that you are supposed to consume in order to be healthy and lean.

But what quantity of those foods are you supposed to eat? Below is a breakdown of the quantities that you are supposed to consume from each of the categories on the pyramid.

What Your Menu Should Have on Daily Basis

- One or two servings of fruits per meal. You can use that as your dessert.

- One or two servings per meal preferably at lunch and dinner of vegetables. It can be nice if one of your servings can contain raw vegetables.

- Four to six servings of healthy fats in a day. One of the most important healthy fats is olive oil, which is a must have because of its high nutritional quality.

- One to three servings of legumes and nuts.

- One or two servings of dairy products like cheese and low-fat yogurt. They are good for strong bones and overall health.

- 1.5 to 2 liters of water. Stay hydrated throughout the day.

- 4-6 servings of whole grains and cereals in the form of couscous, rice, pasta and bread per day.

- 1 glass of wine if you are a woman and 2 glasses of wine if you are a man due to the differences in body weight.

- 30 minutes or more of physical exercises every day. I can't emphasize this enough. It has helped me to lose and then stabilize at my ideal weight, especially going for a brisk. I feel a lot better and refreshed after I exercise.

What Your Menu Should Have on Weekly Basis

- Two to three servings of fish and other seafood

- Two to four servings of eggs

- One to three servings of poultry.

What Your Menu Should Have on A Monthly Basis;

- Red meats like lamb, veal and beef should be eaten only three to four times every month. Buy grass fed meats where possible but I know it is more expensive.

- Sweets should only be eaten 2-3 times in a month. Again, I think if you do this moderation, it will be fine and keep you from wanted to have them more often.

Step 3: Go for Shopping

The Mediterranean Diet is mostly about a lifestyle of eating.

For you to eat, you will need to first have some food to cook. So, the third step is for you to go out and shop for healthy groceries that are Mediterranean friendly. But before you do that, you need to first cleanse your kitchen by donating or throwing out any food that is not Mediterranean friendly.

After that, you will need to make a shopping list that will guide you on what to buy when you go grocery shopping. So how does a shopping list look like?

Check out an example of one below:

Sample Shopping List and Suggested Servings (with Moderation and Smaller Portions)

Vegetables – Daily Servings – 1 to 2 Per Meal

( ) Asparagus   ( ) Cauliflower   ( ) Mushrooms

( ) Avocado	( ) Green Beans	( ) Onions
( ) Broccoli	( ) Mushrooms	( ) Potatoes
( ) Brussel Sprouts	( ) Green Bell Peppers	( ) Spinach
( ) Carrots	( ) Kale	( ) Squash

Fruits – Daily Servings – 1 to 2 Per Meal (Moderation Due to Sugar)

( ) Apples	( ) Cranberries	( ) Raspberries
( ) Bananas	( ) Kiwis	( ) Red Grapes
( ) Blackberries	( ) Olives	( ) Strawberries
( ) Blueberries	( ) Oranges	( ) Tomatoes
( ) Cantaloupes	( ) Papayas	

Whole Grains, Bread, and Pasta – Daily Servings – 4 to 6 Servings

| ( ) Brown Rice | ( ) Quinoa | ( ) Whole Grain Pastas |
| ( ) Oatmeal | ( ) Whole Grain Breads | ( ) Other Whole Grain Products |

Legumes (Beans) – Daily Servings – 1 to 3 Servings

| ( ) Black Beans | ( ) Kidney Beans | ( ) Peas |
| ( ) Garbanzo Beans | ( ) Lentils | ( ) Pinto Beans |

Nuts – Daily Servings – 1 to 3 Servings (Moderation Due to High Calories)

| ( ) Almonds | ( ) Hazelnuts | ( ) Pistachios |
| ( ) Brazil Nuts | ( ) Macadamia Nuts | ( ) Walnuts |

( ) Cashews   ( ) Pecans

Eggs, Cheese, Poultry, Yogurt, Vegetarian – Daily to Weekly Servings

( ) Chicken Breasts   ( ) Greek Yogurt   ( ) Seitan

( ) Eggs - Free Range   ( ) Mozzarella Cheese   ( ) Tofu / Soy Products

( ) Feta Cheese   ( ) Parmesan Cheese   ( ) Turkey

Fish (Wild Where Feasible), Seafood – A Few Times Per Week

( ) Haddock   ( ) Shellfish – Mussels,   ( ) Tuna
                     Oysters

( ) Salmon   ( ) Shrimp, Crab and
                     Lobster

Meat and Sweets – Monthly or in Small Amounts

( ) Red Meat – Grass Fed   ( ) Sweets – for your sweet
                            tooth

Oils – As Required and in Moderation

( ) Extra Virgin Olive Oil   ( ) Grapeseed Oil

This is a perfect example of a good shopping list. Make one for yourself and use it to shop. Once you are done, hung the list on your fridge and use it to check off the supplies that you have run out of in the course of the week. This will make your life easier because it will help you know what you have and what you don't have.

Step 4: Cook

The culture of Mediterranean Diet advocates for people to cook for themselves. This is because the process of cooking usually relaxes you and gives you pleasure, two factors that promote your health. Therefore, find some good recipes and get creative as you prepare them in the kitchen. The last chapter of this book is going to provide you with easy to make recipes that you can prepare over the next 30 days or more.

Step 5: Make a Goal of Sitting Down with Family When Eating

Countries around the Mediterranean Sea have a culture where meals are often consumed in the company of family and friends. They consider meal times as a time of pleasure with family and friends.

That's why the fifth step is for you to try your best to be eating with your family or friends during meal times. I know this can be difficult due to everyone's busy schedules but try to do it as often as you can. I usually have to reserve a couple of nights to make sure we eat together at least twice a week. It may be easier to do this over a weekend.

Why is this important?

Well, eating with company is usually important because it helps you not to overeat. When you eat with family and friends, you tend to be more joyful and more relaxed. That makes you eat slowly thus enabling you to know when you are full and when to stop eating.

Step 6: Exercise

As you saw previously, exercise is an essential part of the Mediterranean diet. In fact, in the updated Mediterranean pyramid, exercising is placed at the bottom or the foundation of the pyramid indicating just how important it is to the Mediterranean diet.

Therefore, the sixth step to starting a Mediterranean diet is to become physically active through exercising. Taking a walk every morning or maybe during lunch or during a break will do wonders.

Before you know what exercises to do when on a Mediterranean Diet, it's important for you to understand why exercising is a crucial part of the Mediterranean Diet.

There are two reasons why exercising is important:

1. It increases your lifespan

   This might come as a surprise to you but the combination of a Mediterranean style of eating and exercising can actually add some years to your life. According to a research that was carried out by Professor Lee, an assistant professor at The State University of Iowa, exercising and more specifically running lowers the rate of premature death by 43 percent. This adds you approximately over 3 years of life with everyone hour of jogging adding you 7 more hours of existence. I prefer walking and hate running.

2. It speeds up your weight loss

When you exercise, your body usually uses up all your readily available energy from dietary glucose and glycogen. This then forces your body to tap into your stored fat in order to match the energy required. This process normally burns down your body fats, which automatically speeds your weight loss.

The question often is what exercises are you supposed to do when on a Mediterranean Diet?

The best exercises to do when on a Mediterranean Diet (or for any diet for that matter) include the following: jogging, running, swimming and long-distance walking. These exercises are good because they increase the rate of your heart beat, which does more to improve your heart health than anything else. The above exercises are also good for you if you are one of those people who don't like paying for gym memberships or buying exercising equipment. This is me!

That said, you can also do other types of exercises like strength training, yoga, calisthenics exercises and aerobics when you are on a Mediterranean Diet. If you find exercising a bit boring for you, then you can do fun exercising activities on a regular basis.

Some of these fun exercising activities include: enrolling for some dance classes, going on a hike, playing with your kids every day, joining your community soccer, basketball or baseball team, and biking with your friends or family.

The information above are the 6 steps that you need to follow to start following a Mediterranean Diet and that will help you get to weight loss goals including a much healthier lifestyle. They are as easy as they look.

Now that you know what to do to start a Mediterranean Diet, what is left is for you to learn some tips that will help you succeed on the diet as a beginner. The next chapter is going to highlight these tips.

Tips of How to Succeed on a Mediterranean Diet

As you now know by now, the Mediterranean Diet is very beneficial. However, not all the people who try it out get the benefits they wanted from it.

One of the reasons why this happens is because most people are never mindful of whose advice they take. In the process, they end up getting misleading information that makes it hard for them to succeed in this diet.

In this chapter, you will learn tips from experienced experts on what you can do to succeed on the Mediterranean diet. The tips will be divided into two sections.

The first set of tips will advice you on what you can do to make the diet less of a challenge and more of a lifestyle that you live your life around. The second set of tips will talk about what you can do in order to improve your success rate on the Mediterranean diet.

Let's look at each of this set of tips below.

How to Make the Diet Feel Less Like a Challenge

- Snack on low fat-cheese, seeds and nuts instead of processed snacks

If you love snacking, you might view the Mediterranean Diet as a challenge for you because it limits your rate of snacking on foods loaded with sugar and saturated fats like cookies and candy. However, you don't have to stop snacking completely, as the Mediterranean Diet allows you to snack on healthy snacks like sunflower seeds, walnuts, low-fat cheese and nonfat plain yogurt.

This means you don't have to change your lifestyle of snacking; you only need to change it and make it healthy.

- Use fruits as your dessert (but in moderation)

As you know by now, the Mediterranean Diet prohibits sugary stuff, which form a big part of the desserts you probably like as I do. Well, that doesn't mean you cannot take care of your sweet tooth.

You can still have your dessert because the diet allows you to eat fruits which can make a good dessert. So, you don't have to give up your love for dessert when you are on the diet. My only recommendation you have noticed is I mention "in moderation". This is key for your long-term success.

- Replace red meat with other proteins like turkey, fish and chicken

Most lovers of red meat find the Mediterranean Diet very challenging for them. This is because the red meat consumption is usually limited to 2-3 times per month. However, you can make it less challenging by switching to other delicious forms of protein like a skinless chicken, fatty fish and turkey.

- Replace the use of butter with olive oil

If you love using margarine and butter for cooking and baking, you don't have to change your lifestyle too much just because they are both prohibited by a Mediterranean Diet. This is because you can replace them with heart healthy oils like extra virgin olive oil, walnut oil and canola oil. You can season them with balsamic vinegar and make a delicious dipping that you can use when eating bread.

Note: Just because I have stated that you should minimize butter doesn't mean you avoid it altogether. You can use it but in moderation.

- Feel free to spice your food

Mediterranean people love spices. You too shouldn't be left behind. In fact, I would greatly recommend that you replace salt (this does not mean you should avoid it altogether) with dried or fresh spices and herbs.

You can also season your food using dried chilies or citrus. You can also use black pepper, thyme, fennel seeds, herbs de Provence, oregano, and whole grated nutmeg.

General Tips of How to Succeed on The Mediterranean Diet

- Have your meals with family and friends. Don't eat alone.

When you eat with your family members or your friends, you usually tend to have a less stressful time and an improved mood, which is good for your overall health. Eating with company also enables you to control the portions of your meal, which helps you not to overeat. As you are well aware, overeating can be recipe for failure in any weight loss diet.

- Always eat breakfast

One of the reasons why most people are not successful on the Mediterranean Diet is because they do not eat breakfast. The truth is that not eating breakfast affects your progress because it means you are likely to have full blown hunger pains before noon. This might in turn make you want to binge eat or overeat, a phenomenon that might result in weight gain.

For you to be successful on the diet, you need to eat a well-balanced breakfast. This will help you stay satisfied for long, give you energy throughout the day, and it will reduce how much food you eat during the course of the day. This will in turn help you to lose weight faster and more efficiently.

- Eat homemade foods

A lot of us today eat out at lunch and at dinner because our tight schedules normally can't allow us to cook something for ourselves. What you need to realize is that for you to be successful on the Mediterranean Diet, you need to put a stop to eating out all the time. Eating out occasionally is fine. I need to.

The restaurants dishes are usually loaded with fats and salt and have a high caloric content, which affect your weight loss and overall health progress. What you should do if you don't have time to cook for yourself every day is to schedule a day that you are free, probably on a Sunday afternoon, and then pre-cook Mediterranean friendly foods for the week.

Store them in the freezer and warm them up whenever you want to eat. If you are going to work, carry a packed lunch. In this way, you will enjoy success because you will have followed the diet strictly. It also helps you to create discipline as part of your new lifestyle.

- Take your time when eating

According to a research that was done in the University of Rhode Island, it takes about 20 minutes for your stomach to alert your brain that it is full. I have experimented with this and stopped eating before I was full. Within 15-20 minutes, I actually felt full and glad I did not keep eating.

So, if you eat too fast, you will easily overeat because your stomach is slow at delivering the message that it's full. The best thing for you to do to make sure that you hardly overeat is to take your time when eating. You can do this by chewing about 10 times before swallowing. This will help you get the 'I am satisfied' message at the right time.

- Drink a lot of water

Water is usually good because of two things. For starters, it fills up your stomach, which makes you take in fewer calories (water has zero calories) when eating, which in turn enables you to lose weight faster.

Secondly, when you drink a lot of water, you tend to lose more weight because your body does not retain water weight like it does when you don't drink enough water. That's why you need to make drinking water a top priority.

- Always place food away from where you are eating

One of the reasons why most people fail when they are on a Mediterranean Diet is because they usually tempt themselves by keeping extra food or the wrong food within their eyesight. This makes you want to reach out for a second helping, which easily turns into overeating and subsequent weight gain.
To ensure this never happens, ensure to always place food on the kitchen counter or anywhere out of your sight when eating. That way, you will limit the temptation to overeat and increase your success while on the diet.

- Eat fiber rich vegetables throughout the day

Nutritionists recommend that we all ought to eat at least 3-8 servings of fruits and vegetables. The Mediterranean Diet is no exception.

Unfortunately, many of us hardly get enough of these. Since a serving ranges between ½ cup to 2 cups depending on the nature of the vegetable, it is important to find ways of ensuring that you eat at least the minimum amount of these to bring about various benefits that come with taking sufficient amounts of veggies.

This is especially important since veggies are high in antioxidants, and various critical vitamins that you need enough of to stay healthy. To ensure you take in enough of fruits and veggies, ensure to start your day with such veggies like carrots (roasted are good), spinach and cheddar omelet, avocado, etc. The idea here is to ensure you have at least as many variety of colored veggies as possible given that each color brings with it various benefits due to different properties.

Feel free to drink smoothies, salads and deliberately include veggies in your meals. I find smoothies are the easiest way for me to get the required number of vegetable servings and often I add fruit.

- Insist on eating whole, organic foods

The Mediterranean region population who lived 50-70 years ago didn't rely heavily on store bought ingredients that were heavily processed. They obtained their ingredients from their local farmer's markets and obtained many others from their farms.

You too shouldn't rely on store bought ingredients especially those processed. Anything that comes in a package with lots of strange set of ingredients should be avoided at all costs.

Following the above tips will undoubtedly increase your chances of succeeding while on the Mediterranean Diet. That said, there are many questions that you will have once you start following the diet.

Below is a list of frequently asked questions chapter that will answer some of the questions that most beginners have when they get started on the Mediterranean Diet.

Frequently Asked Questions

In this chapter, we are going to look at some frequent asked questions about the Mediterranean Diet and their answers. Check them out below.

Q: What Is the Difference Between a Mediterranean Diet and A Low Carb Diet?

A: A low carb diet and a Mediterranean Diet are usually quite similar. Their only major difference is the protein content that they advocate. In a low carb diet, you are supposed to get 25-30% of your calorie intake from proteins while in a Mediterranean Diet, you are only recommended to consume about 15% of your daily calorie from proteins.

Q: What Is the Difference Between the American Diet and The Mediterranean Diet?

A: There are many differences between the typical American diet and the Mediterranean Diet but the two major differences are the ingredients used in both diets and the frequency you can consume the ingredients.

For instance, the American diet allows you to eat saturated fats like margarine and butter while the Mediterranean diet forbids you from eating majority of the saturated fats. However, that doesn't mean you cannot use such ingredients like butter. What you need to do is to be very deliberate about moderating your intake of these ingredients.

In fact, if you don't want to use them, you are free to replace them with healthier alternatives like olive oil and other allowed fats. The two diets allow you to eat meat, eggs, sweets and poultry products but the Mediterranean Diet limits your consumption to only one or two times in a week while the American diet allows you to consume them as frequently as you would like.

Q: How Much Fat Should You Consume When on A Mediterranean Diet?

A: The ideal amount of fat to consume when you are on a Mediterranean Diet is about 30% of your calorie intake. However, you should make sure that only one third or less than 10% of those fats come from saturated fats like fatty meats. As you noticed (in the Mediterranean Diet pyramid), fatty meats are supposed to only be consumed occasionally or a few times in a month.

Q: Is It Possible for You to Calculate the Fat Percentage from A Packaged Food Item?

A: The answer is yes. Almost all packaged food items have a nutrition fact label that indicates the amount of fat calories per serving, fat and saturated fat grams per servings. Here is how to calculate the fat percentage:

You will first need to know the fat calories per serving. If it's not indicated in the label, you can calculate it by multiplying the number of saturated fat or fat grams in a serving by 9

For example, if you have a low-fat plain yogurt that has been indicated to have 200 calories and 4 grams of fat, you can get the fat calories by multiply 4 grams by 9 to get 36 calories of fat.

The second step is for you to divide the number of calories from fat by the total number of calories per servings. According to our above example, our number of calories of fat is 36 and the total number of calories per servings is 200. So, divide 36 by 200 to get approximately 6.

That means the percentage of fat in the yogurt is 6 percent.

Q: Is It a Must to Consume Wine When on A Mediterranean Diet?

A: The answer is no. Wine is optional. You can achieve your weight loss goals and optimum health without it. But if you do drink wine, do it in moderation.

Q: What Words Suggest You Want a Low-Fat Meal When You Are Eating Out?

A: The best way to order a low-fat dish is to ask for baked, broiled, grilled, stir-fried and sautéed meals. Some restaurants also allow you to make a specific cooking suggestion like telling them to prepare your meal with olive oil or you tell them to cook your meal with minimal oil.

Those are some of the questions that people ask when they are on a Mediterranean Diet. With what we have learned in mind, our next step will be to learn how to cook the Mediterranean way.

30-Day Easy to Cook Recipes

As a beginner, the Mediterranean diet can be a bit challenging especially given that you might not be used to the majority of Mediterranean friendly foods. That will automatically make it difficult for you to cook and prepare your meals. But you shouldn't be worried about that because this chapter is going to provide you with 30 days of recipes that you can use to prepare breakfast, lunch and dinner. Let's begin.

Delicious Mediterranean Breakfast Recipes

Below are some of the best breakfast recipes:

1. Greek Vegetable and Cheese Pie

Prep Time: 35 Minutes, Cook Time: 40 Minutes, Total Time: 75 Minutes

Serves 6

Calories: 252, Fat: 9g, Carbohydrates: 31g, Proteins: 13g

Ingredients

½ cup of crumbled feta cheese with reduced-fat

10 sheets of thawed frozen phyllo dough (14x9 inch)

Nonstick cooking spray

1/8 teaspoon of ground nutmeg

A quarter teaspoon of freshly grounded black pepper

¼ teaspoon of salt

2 lightly beaten eggs

1 ½ cups of evaporated low-fat milk

¼ teaspoon of salt

2 cloves of minced garlic

1 10-ounce package of chopped, thawed and well drained spinach

2 ½ cups of 2 medium thinly sliced zucchini

¾ cup of 1 medium red sweet pepper chopped

1 cup of chopped onions

1 tablespoon of olive oil

Directions

Start by preheating your oven to 375 degrees F.

Use a nonstick skillet to heat oil over medium-high heat. Add in sweet pepper and onion. Cook them until the vegetable is tender or for about 4 minutes. Add in the zucchini and let it cook until it starts to brown. That will take about 4 minutes. Add in ¼ teaspoon of salt, garlic and spinach. Let everything cook for 2 minutes.

Combine the black pepper, ¼ teaspoon salt, eggs, evaporated milk and nutmeg in a small bowl.

Prepare a 9-inch pie plate by coating it with cooking spray. Then spread out the phyllo dough and remove one sheet of the dough. Cover the rest of the phyllo dough to prevent it from drying out. Position the phyllo dough into the prepared pie plate and then light coat it with cooking spray.

Gently press the phyllo dough into the bottom of the pie plate. Do the same on the up sides of the pie plate and let the phyllo sheet ends hang over the edges of the pie plate. Repeat the whole process with the remaining phyllo sheets. Use a crisscross pattern to place the sheets.

Next, evenly spoon the vegetable mixture that you made earlier over the phyllo. Then sprinkle the feta cheese over the vegetables and then pour egg mixture on top. Fold up the overlapping ends of the phyllo towards the center of the pie plate. Now coat the phyllo top with cooking oil as you gently press the pie so that it can hold its shape.

Place the pie on the oven and bake for 40 minutes or until it comes out clean if you insert a folk.

Place on a wire rack to let it cool (for about 15 minutes) then cut it into wedges and serve while warm.

2. Zucchini and Tomato Frittata

Prep Time: 10 Minutes, Cook Time: 20 Minutes, Total Time: 30 Minutes

Serves 4

Calories: 281, Fat: 22g, Carbohydrates: 4g, Proteins: 17g

Ingredients

1/3 cup of coarsely chopped walnuts

2 ounces of bite-size boccoccini (fresh mozzarella balls)

½ cup of halved red and yellow cherry tomatoes

1 small thinly sliced (lengthwise) zucchini

1 tablespoon of olive oil

¼ teaspoon of crushed red pepper

¼ teaspoon of salt

8 eggs

Directions

Start by preheating the broiler and then whisk crushed red pepper, salt and eggs together in a medium bowl.

In a 10-inch oven-usable skillet, heat olive oil over medium-high heat.

Next, evenly layer zucchini slices at the bottom of the skillet then let them cook for about 3 minutes. Turn them only once.

Then top with the cherry tomatoes before pouring in the egg mixture and top that off with walnuts and mozzarella balls. Let them cook over medium heat until the sides begin to set. This should take 4 to 5 minutes. Occasionally lift with a spatula to enable the uncooked portion to run underneath.

Broil the frittata 4 inches from the heat until set or for about 2 to 3 minutes. Next, cut the frittata into wedges then serve.

3. Egg Tartine And Artichoke

Prep Time: 2 Minutes, Cook Time: 13 Minutes, Total Time: 15 Minutes

Serves 1

Calories: 314, Fat: 16g, Carbohydrates: 23g, Proteins: 19g

Ingredients

2 poached or fried large eggs

1 slice of whole-wheat toasted bread

1/8 teaspoon of ground pepper

¼ teaspoon of dried oregano

1 slice of scallion

½ cup of thawed frozen artichoke hearts that are finely chopped

1 teaspoon of extra virgin olive oil

Directions

Start by heating olive oil in a small skillet until hot.

Add in artichoke hearts, pepper, oregano and scallion. Sauté until they are hot.

Then spread the artichoke mixture on toast and then top it off with the eggs.

Serve and enjoy.

4. Almond-Date Smoothie

Prep Time: 10 Minutes, Total Time: 10 Minutes

Serves 2

Calories: 429, Fat: 12g, Carbohydrates: 20g, Proteins: 6g

Ingredients

1 cup of ice cubes

2 tablespoons of almond butter

1 small banana

½ cup of pitted medjool dates

1½ cups of unsweetened almond milk

2 tablespoons

Directions

Place the dates in a heatproof bowl and cover them with boiling water for about 10 minutes. Drain the dates and let them cool. Alternatively, combine the dates and almond milk in a medium bowl. Cover and let them chill overnight.

Use a blender to combine the dates, almond butter, banana and milk. Cover the blender and pulse for about 30 seconds or until the mixture is smooth.

Add in the ice cubes and blend for another 10 seconds.

Pour the mixture into a glass and enjoy.

5. Egg Scramble with Spinach and Cherry Tomatoes

Prep Time: 5 Minutes, Cook Time: 20 Minutes, Total Time: 25 Minutes

Serves 4

Calories: 142, Fat: 6g, Carbohydrates: 7g, Proteins: 15g

Ingredients

¼ cup of finely shredded parmesan cheese

2 cups of halved cherry tomatoes

2 cups packed fresh baby spinach

1 clove of minced garlic

1 tablespoon of olive oil

¼ teaspoon of ground black pepper

½ teaspoon of salt

½ cup of light cream milk

12 thawed egg whites

Directions

Use a medium bowl to combine pepper, salt, milk and egg whites. Whisk the mixture until well mixed and set aside.

Next, heat the olive oil over medium high heat using a large nonstick skillet. Add in garlic and let it cook for 30 seconds as you occasionally stir. Add tomatoes and spinach and let them cook for a further 1 minute as you occasionally stir. The tomatoes should be softened and the spinach wilted at the end of 1 minute. Remove the mixture from the skillet and keep warm.

Transfer the egg white mixture into the skillet and cook over medium heat. Do not stir the mixture; just let it cook until it starts to set on the bottom and on the edges.

Use a large spoon or a spatula to lift and fold the partly cooked egg to allow the uncooked portion to flow underneath. Continue cooking the egg until it is thoroughly cooked but still moist and glossy. This should take you 2 to 3 minutes (ensure it is still moist and glossy). Remove the egg white mixture from heat then top it with the spinach mixture before sprinkling with cheese.

6. Cinnamon French Toast

Prep Time: 5 Minutes, Cook Time: 15 Minutes, Total Time: 20 Minutes

Serves 2

Calories: 281, Fat: 10.8 g, Carbohydrates: 37.2g, Proteins: 14.5g

Ingredients

1 tablespoon of olive oil

4 slices of sprouted cinnamon raisin whole grain bread

1 teaspoon of vanilla extract

1 teaspoon of ground cinnamon

½ cup of unsweetened almond milk

2 eggs

Directions

Start by combining vanilla, cinnamon, almond milk and eggs in a shallow bowl. Use a fork to whip them together until well combined.

Then add the bread slices into your prepared egg mixture and let them soak for 2 minutes.

Next, heat the olive oil in a skillet over medium-high heat. Add in the soaked bread and cook it until golden brown or for about 1 to 2 minutes on every side. Place the toast on a serving plate.

Serve the toast with a sprinkle of cinnamon, maple syrup and enjoy.

7. Potato Hash and Chickpea

Prep Time: 5 Minutes, Cook Time: 20 Minutes, Total Time: 25 Minutes

Serves 4

Calories: 382, Fat: 20g, Carbohydrates: 37, Proteins: 14g

Ingredients

4 large eggs

1 cup of chopped zucchini

1 15 ounce rinsed can chickpeas

¼ cup extra-virgin olive oil

½ teaspoon of salt

1 tablespoon of curry powder

1 tablespoon of minced fresh ginger

½ cup of finely chopped onion

2 cups of finely chopped baby spinach

4 cups of frozen hash brown potatoes, shredded

Directions

Start by combining salt, curry powder, ginger, onion, spinach and potatoes in a large bowl.

Use a large nonstick skillet to heat oil over medium-high heat. Pour in the potato mixture and force it down into a layer. Let it cook without stirring until it turns golden brown on the bottom and is crisp. This should take you 3 to 5 minutes.

Decrease the heat to medium-low heat and then fold in zucchini and chickpeas while ensuring potato chunks break up nicely until very nicely combined. Next, press them nicely to form an even layer then carve out 4 wells into the mixture.

Next, break each egg, one at a time, into a cup. Then pour them into each 'well'. Cover the skillet and let everything cook for 4 to 5 minutes.

Serve on a plate and enjoy.

8. Mediterranean Frittata

Prep Time: 5 Minutes, Cook Time: 20 Minutes, Total Time: 25 Minutes

Serves 6

Calories: 246, Fat: 19g, Carbohydrates: 8g, Proteins: 11g

Ingredients

Fresh basil leaves

2 tablespoons of parmesan, finely shredded parmesan

½ cup of onion and garlic croutons, coarsely crushed.

1/8 teaspoon of ground black pepper

¼ cup of slivered fresh basil

½ cup of pitted ripe olives or sliced kalamata

½ cup of chopped and roasted red sweet peppers. Bottled

½ cup of crumbled feta cheese

¼ cup of half and half

8 beaten eggs

3 tablespoons of olive oil

2 cloves of minced garlic

1 cup of chopped onion

Directions

Start by preheating the broiler.

Heat 2 tablespoons of oil in a broiler proof skillet and add in onion and garlic. Let them cook until the onion is tender.

As the onion cooks, beat the eggs and half and half together in a bowl. Stir in black pepper, basil, olives, roasted sweet pepper and feta cheese.

Then pour the egg mixture on top of the onions in the broiler proof skillet. Let the mixture cook over medium heat.

Use a spatula to run on the edges of the mixture once it starts to set. Lift the mixture with the spatula and let the uncooked portion to flow underneath. Reduce heat and continue cooking until the egg mixture is thoroughly cooked but still moist on the surface.

Use a bowl to combine the remaining tablespoons of oil, parmesan cheese, and crushed croutons until well combined. Sprinkle the mixture on top of the frittata.

Broil the frittata for 1 to 2 minutes, 5 inches from the heat. The crumbs should be golden and the top set after the 2 minutes. Slice the frittata into wedges and serve on a plate. Garnish with fresh basil leaves and enjoy.

9. Mediterranean Nut Banana Oatmeal

Prep Time: 5 Minutes, Cook Time: 2 Minutes, Total Time: 7 Minutes

Serves 1

Calories: 425, Fat: 17.5g, Carbohydrates: 62.5g, Proteins: 12.5g

Ingredients

1 peeled banana

3 tablespoons of honey

2 tablespoons of chopped walnuts

1 teaspoon of flax seeds

½ cup of skim milk

¼ cup of quick cooking oats

Directions

Start by combining banana, honey, walnuts, flax seeds, milk and oats in a microwave safe bowl.

Place the bowl in the microwave and let it cook for 2 minutes on high.

Then squash the banana using a fork and then stir it onto the mixture.

Serve on a plate while hot and enjoy.

10. Greek Yogurt Pancake

Prep Time: 5 Minutes, Cook Time: 20 Minutes, Total Time: 25 Minutes

Serves 2

Calories: 225, Fat: 5.5g, Carbohydrates: 25.38g, Proteins: 13.5g

Ingredients

1 teaspoon of baking soda

½ cup of whole wheat pastry flour

2 egg whites or 1 egg

¾ cups of Greek yogurt

2 tablespoons of canola oil

Directions

Start by combining eggs and Greek yogurt in a bowl. Beat them together until creamy.

In another bowl, mix the baking soda and flour.

Then mix the egg (wet) mixture with the flour (dry) mixture until they form a well-combined batter. Let the batter rest for 10 minutes.

Heat the canola oil on a non-stick skillet over medium heat. Pour in a ¼ cup of batter into the skillet.

Cook the pancakes until bubbles start forming on top of the pancake and the bottom is golden brown; this should take 2 minutes. Turn the pancake over and cook the other side until the bottom takes a golden brown color i.e. for about 2 minutes. Repeat this process until you have used up all the batter.

Serve.

11. Kalamata Olives with Mediterranean Style Eggs

Prep Time: 5 Minutes, Cook Time: 15 Minutes, Total Time: 20 Minutes

Serves 3

Calories: 277, Fat: 11g, Carbohydrates: 23g, Proteins: 17g

Ingredients

10 diced Kalamata olives

2 chopped Roma tomatoes

1 15.5 ounce can of organic chickpeas

Cracked pepper

¼ cup of unsweetened vanilla almond milk

5 eggs

1 cup of spinach

Olive oil with lemon or citrus juice (Use plain olive oil and sprinkle lemon juice when cooking if you can't get the infused one)

Directions

Heat up the olive oil infused with lemon in a pan over medium heat. Add in spinach and sauté until it is lightly wilted. This should take you 2 minutes. Remove and place in a medium bowl.

Sprinkle olive oil in the pan that has just sautéed the spinach. In a separate medium sized bowl, mix almond milk and eggs. Heat the pan up and pour in the egg mixture. Season with cracked pepper and let it continue cooking.

Meanwhile, add tomatoes, olives and chickpeas into the spinach bowl and mix everything together.

Toss the spinach mixture into the pan; this should be after the eggs have scrambled to your liking. Season with the remaining cracked pepper.

Transfer the egg mixture on a plate. Serve while hot and enjoy.

12. Oatmeal with Raspberries and Seeds

Cook Time: 20 Minutes, Total Time: 20 Minutes

Serves 2 or 3

Calories: 285, Fat: 10.2g, Carbohydrates: 47.9, Proteins: 16.4g

Ingredients

½ teaspoon of ground cinnamon

1-2 teaspoons of olive oil

Pinch of salt

2 cups of boiling water

1 cup of rolled oats

Toppings

Honey

Seeds or any nuts of your choice

Fresh berries (You can use any fruit)

Directions

Start by cooking the oats; place the oats in a saucepan and add in water and salt. Heat the saucepan to bring the oats to a boil. Let the mixture boil for 5 minutes

Decrease the heat and let the oat mixture simmer for 5-10 minutes as you stir regularly. The water should be absorbed and the oats should be creamy by the end of 10 minutes.

Take the saucepan off the heat. Add in cinnamon and olive oil before covering the saucepan with a lid. Let the mixture steam for 5 minutes.

Give the oats a good stir and then transfer them on to a serving plate. Top them with seeds, berries and a sprinkle of honey. Enjoy.

13. Avocado and Toasted Rye

Prep Time: 5 Minutes, Cook Time: 5 Minutes, Total Time: 10 Minutes

Serves 4

Calories: 1200, Fat: 20, Carbohydrates: 19g, Proteins: 9g

Ingredients

4 large slices of rye bread

A squeeze of lemon juice, fresh

2 tablespoons of fresh mint (chopped) plus an extra mint to garnish

80 grams of crumbled creamy feta

2 peeled firm ripe avocados with the stone removed

Directions

Start by rough mashing the avocado in a medium sized bowl using a fork. Add in a squeeze of lemon juice and mint. Then mash the mixture until well combined.

Season the mixture with freshly ground black pepper and some salt.

Grill or toast the rye bread until golden. Then place it on a plate and use the avocado mixture as topping, top with feta and then garnish with some more mint.

14. Mediterranean Jalapeno and Dill

Prep Time: 20 Minutes, Cook Time: 12 Hours, Total Time: 12 Hours. 20 Minutes

Serves 8

Calories: 87, Fat: 4g, Carbohydrates: 7g, Proteins: 6g

Ingredients

½ teaspoon of cumin seeds

1 tablespoon of chopped fresh parsley

1 tablespoon of chopped fresh dill

1 tablespoon of extra virgin oil

1 small sliced jalapeno pepper

¼ cup of sliced scallions

¼ teaspoon of salt

1 quart of low-fat plain yogurt

Directions

Start by using 4 layers of cheesecloth to line up a large fine-mesh sieve or a 7 inch sieve. Then set the cheesecloth over a bowl that is deep enough to create a 3 inches difference between the bowl and the bottom of the sieve.

In a separate medium sized bowl, beat yogurt with salt then spoon the mixture onto the cheesecloth.

Next, refrigerate the yogurt for 12 to 24 hours; the yogurt should be thick by the time you remove it from the fridge. By this time, about 1 cup of liquid should have drained into the bowl. You can discard this the liquid.

Top the yogurt with cumin seeds, parsley, dill oil, jalapeno and scallions.

Serve.

15. Mediterranean Pizza

Prep Time: 7 Minutes, Cook Time: 10 Minutes, Total Time: 17 Minutes

Serves 4

Calories: 291, Fat: 11g, Carbohydrates: 34g, Proteins: 14g

Ingredients

4 teaspoons of dried basil or ¼ cup of chopped fresh basil

Cooking spray

14 ounce can of drained quartered artichoke hearts

6 chopped pitted kalamata olives

3 slices of plum tomatoes

1 cup of crumbled goat cheese

¼ teaspoon of Italian seasoning, dried

¼ teaspoon of crushed red pepper

1 (12 inch) prepared pizza crust

Directions

Start by preheating your oven to 450 degrees F.

Then use the dried Italian seasoning and crushed red pepper to sprinkle over the pizza crust. Add in crumbled goat cheese by sprinkling it evenly on the crust. Make sure that you leave a ½ inch border.

Gently press down the cheese on the pizza crust; you can use the back of a spoon for that.

Then arrange the quartered artichoke hearts, chopped olives and the plum tomato slices one by one on top of the pizza.

Coat the pizza with cooking spray and place it on the baking sheet. Put the baking sheet inside the oven and bake for 10-12 minutes or until the cheese is bubbly and the crust is crisp.

Remove from the oven and top it with a sprinkle of chopped basil.

Serve while hot.

16. Overnight Oats with Fruits

Prep time: 10 minutes, Freeze time: 6-24 hours

Serves 4

Calories: 530, Fat: 18g, Carbohydrates: 81g, Proteins: 17g

Ingredients

1 cup of fresh raspberries

1, 6 ounce, can of yogurt (choose your desired flavor)

1 seeded, cored and thinly sliced tart green apple

¾ cup of pecans, blanched almonds and toasted and coarsely chopped walnuts

1 teaspoon of ground cinnamon

¼ cup of honey

1 cup of apple juice

1 cup of milk

2 cups of regular rolled oats

Directions

Start by dividing ½ cup of oats into 4 half pint jars (8 ounce).

Use a separate cup to combine cinnamon, honey, apple juice and milk. Pour the mixture on top of the oats in the four jars.

Cover the jars and let them chill overnight or until the oats are soft.

Sprinkle in the nuts and top that off with yogurt and a fruit of your choice like raspberries.

Serve and enjoy.

17. Scrambled Eggs with Spinach & Smoked Trout

Prep Time: 15 Minutes, Total Time: 15 Minutes

Serves 2

Calories: 243, Fat: 17g, Carbohydrates: 4g, Proteins: 19g

Ingredients

1 cup of chopped spinach

½ cup of boned and flaked smoked trout

2 tablespoons of finely chopped shallot

2 teaspoons of avocado or grape seed oil

Pinch of salt

¼ teaspoon of ground pepper

2 tablespoons of reduced fat milk

4 large eggs

Directions

Start by mixing salt, pepper, milk and eggs in a medium bowl. Whisk until the mixture is all pale yellow.

Use a medium nonstick skillet to heat oil over medium heat. Add in shallot and cook until it starts to brown. Stir regularly. This should take you 1 to 2 minutes.

Reduce the heat to medium and then add the egg mixture. Let the mixture cook undisturbed for about 30 seconds or until it starts to set on the edges.

Toss the trout over the eggs and start to gently push and fold the eggs with a spatula until they are fluffy but hardly set. That should take 2 to 4 minutes.

Then add in the spinach, stir well and then remove the skillet from the heat. Put a lid on the skillet and let the mixture stand for 1 or 2 minutes or until the spinach is wilted.

Transfer the scrambled egg mixture onto a serving plate and serve while hot.

18. Mediterranean Tahini-feta toast

Prep Time: 8 Minutes, Cook Time: 10 Minutes, Total Time: 18 Minutes

Serves 2

Calories: 180, Fat: 9g, Carbohydrates: 19g, Proteins: 7g

Ingredients

Pepper

2 teaspoons of pine nuts

2 teaspoons of crumbled feta

1 teaspoon of water

Juice from ½ lemon

1 tablespoon of tahini

2 slices of whole wheat bread

Directions

Start by preparing tahini. Combine lemon juice, water and tahini in a small bowl and mix until everything is well combined. The consistency should be thick but not as thick as a peanut butter (it should be easy to spread). In case yours is too thick, you can add a bit of water and make it just slightly thick.

Then toast the bread. This should take you 5 to 10 minutes.

Next, spread the tahini mixture on the toasted bread then top this with the crumbled feta and pine nuts.

Add some pepper to taste and serve.

19. Mediterranean Macaroni and Cheese

Prep Time: 10 Minutes, Cook Time: 50 Minutes, Total Time: 1 Hr.

Serves 6

Calories: 392.3, Fat: 16.8g, Carbohydrates: 46.8g, Proteins: 15.9g

Ingredients

Freshly grounded black pepper and salt to taste

½ cup of panko bread crumbs

2 ounce of shredded mozzarella cheese

6 ounce of crumbled feta cheese

2 cups of low fat milk

3 tablespoons of all-purpose flour

¼ teaspoon of granulated garlic

1/3 cup of chopped red onion

2 tablespoons of extra virgin oil

8 ounce of tri color rotini pasta

1 tablespoon of Mediterranean dry rub

1 tablespoon of chopped fresh basil (have some more for garnish)

1/3 cup of chopped pitted kalamata olives

1 can (14.5 oz.) of low sodium tomatoes, diced and drained

Directions

Start by preheating your oven to 400 degrees F and then lightly brush an 8 by 8 inch baking dish with olive oil. Set the baking dish aside.

Mix the Mediterranean dry rub, basil, chopped olives and drained diced tomatoes in a small mixing bowl. Set the mixture aside.

Prepare the pasta by following the instructions on the package. Ensure reserve about ½ cup of the pasta water then return it to the pot.

Heat up the remaining olive oil in a saucepan over medium heat. Add in onions and sauté them for 3-4 minutes or until soft and lightly golden. During the last minute of sautéing, add in granulated garlic. Next, whisk in the flour and stir continually for 1 minute as it cooks. Slowly pour in the milk as you stir ensuring to break up any flour lumps. Bring the mixture to a boil while regularly stirring the mixture.

Decrease the heat to medium low and simmer (immediately the mixture reaches a boil). Continue stirring for about 3 minutes or until the mixture has thickened. Remove the saucepan from the heat and stir in mozzarella and feta cheese. Season the sauce with pepper and salt to taste.

Transfer the tomato mixture that you made earlier over the drained pasta and give it a toss. Pour in the sauce that you have just made over the pasta mixture and toss for it to evenly coat. Add the reserved pasta water if the mixture is a bit dry.

Transfer the pasta mixture onto the prepared baking dish. Next, sprinkle the pasta mixture with panko and feta cheese as toppings.

Place the baking dish on the oven and bake for 20-25 minutes or until the top turns golden brown.

Serve the pasta warm and garnish with fresh basil.

20. Lemon Strawberry Poppy Seed Parfait

Prep Time: 10 Minutes, Total Time: 10 Minutes

Serves 1

Calories: 340, Fat: 11g, Carbohydrates: 49g, Proteins: 14g

Ingredients

1 tablespoon of poppy seeds

1 tablespoon of lemon curd

1 cup of sliced strawberries

1 cup of plain low fat yogurt

Directions

Start by scooping half of the yogurt in a parfait jar or glass.

Then top the yogurt with half of the lemon curd, half of the poppy seeds and lastly half of the strawberries. Repeat the whole process again for the second time.

Serve and enjoy.

21. Mediterranean Green Bean Casserole

Prep Time: 10 Minutes, Cook Time: 20 Minutes, Total Time: 30 Minutes

Serves 8

Calories: 176, Fat: 13g, Carbohydrates: 11g, Proteins: 6g

Ingredients

½ cup of shredded sharp cheddar cheese

1 cup of cherry tomatoes

¼ cup of extra virgin olive oil

½ teaspoon of salt

¾ teaspoon of ground cumin

1 small clove garlic

1 tablespoon of lime juice

1-3 tablespoons of chopped jalapeno pepper

½ cup of divided roasted shelled pistachios

½ cup of fresh herbs like chopped chives, parsley and cilantro

2 pounds of trimmed and cut into 2 pieces green beans

Directions

Start by putting water in a large pot then bring it to a boil. Then add in the green beans and let them cook for 4-6 minutes or until they are crisp and tender. Drain the beans and rinse with cold water.

Preheat your broiler to a high after you've positioned a rack in the upper third of the oven.

Use a food processor to mix salt, cumin, garlic, lime juice, jalapeno to taste, herbs and ¼ cup of pistachios. Beat the mixture until everything is finely chopped as you scrap the sides once or twice. Add oil as the food processor is processing. Make sure everything is well combined. This should take you not more than 5 minutes.

Dry the green beans and place them on a 9 by 13 inch broiler safe pan. Add tomatoes and sauce into the pan and toss well to combine. Then sprinkle the cheese on the beans.

Broil the casserole for 4-6 minutes or until the cheese has melted and starts to brown. Chop the ¼ cup pistachios that remained and sprinkle over the top.

Serve and enjoy.

22. Banana and Mango Smoothie

Prep Time: 5 Minutes, Cook Time: 1 Hour, Total Time: 1 Hour 5 Min

Serves 2

Calories: 168, Fat: 1g, Carbohydrates: 39g, Proteins: 4g

Ingredients

4-6 ice cubes

½ cup of unsweetened almond milk or skim milk

½ cup of beet juice

1 small mango

1 frozen pre sliced banana

½ inch slice of fresh ginger root

2 cups of loosely packed organic baby spinach

Directions

Start by washing the beets and patting them dry. Then proceed to preheat the oven to 375 degrees F.

Apply and rub olive oil on the outside part of the beets. Then wrap the beets in a foil and roast them for 50-60 minutes or until they are tender. Let them cool and then peel.

Toss the beets and all the above ingredients in a blender and then blend until smooth.

Pour the smoothie into a glass. Serve and enjoy.

23. Cheese Pies-Tyropita

Prep Time: 8 Hour 15 Minutes, Cook Time: 20 Minutes, Total Time: 8 Hour 35 Minutes

Serves 2

Calories: 320, Fat: 25g, Carbohydrates: 19g, Proteins: 10g

Ingredients

1 package phyllo

Olive oil

Pepper

1 cup of chopped fresh mint

2 eggs

2 tablespoon of Greek style yogurt

3 tablespoons of low fat cream cheese

1 ounce of feta grams

8 ounce of anthotyro or ricotta

Directions

Start by preheating the oven to 350 degrees F.

Use a small bowl to grind the feta with a fork. Then whisk the eggs in another separate small bowl.

Combine mint, pepper, eggs and cheeses in a large bowl. Mix them together until well combined. Let the mixture sit overnight or for a few hours.

To make the tyropitakia, defrost the phyllo and spread out 1 sheet. Brush olive oil on the sheet and cut it into 4 strips lengthwise.

Place 1½ teaspoons of cheese mixture at the top corner of each strip. Start folding each strip in a small triangle. Repeat the process until the whole mixture has been used up.

Rest the cheese pies in an already light greased pan. Brush the pies with a small amount of olive oil.

Put the pies on the oven and let them bake for 20 minutes or until golden.

Remove from the oven and let them cool. Serve and enjoy.

24. Mediterranean Vegetable Omelet

Prep Time: 15 Minutes, Cook Time: 25 Minutes, Total Time: 40 Minutes

Serves 4

Calories: 152, Fat: 10g, Carbohydrates: 6g, Proteins: 11g

Ingredients

2 tablespoons of dill, parsley or basil

½ cup of crumbled goat cheese

½ teaspoon of pepper

¼ teaspoon of salt

6 eggs

¼ cup of artichoke hearts (Should be marinated in water, rinsed, drained and chopped)

¼ cup of chopped pitted green brine-cured olives.

1 Roma tomato, diced

2 cups of thinly sliced fresh fennel bulb

1 tablespoon of olive oil

Directions

Start by preheating the oven to 325 degrees F.

Next, heat the olive oil using a large ovenproof skillet over medium high heat. Add in the fennel and sauté until soft. This should take you 5 minutes.

Add in artichoke hearts, olives and tomato then sauté the mixture for 3 minutes.

Meanwhile, crack the eggs and pour on a large bowl. Whisk the eggs and season them with some salt and pepper. Add the eggs into the vegetable skillet and stir for about 2 minutes using a heatproof spoon.

Sprinkle some cheese on top of the omelet and place the mixture on the oven to bake for 5 minutes.

Top the omelet with dill, parsley or basil before removing it from the skillet and placing it on a cutting board.

Cut the omelet into four edges and serve while hot.

25. Almonds Berry Smoothie

Prep Time: 10 Minute, Total Time: 10 Minutes

Serves 1

Calories: 360, Fat: 19g, Carbohydrates: 46g, Proteins: 9g

Ingredients

1 tablespoon of unsweetened coconut flakes

¼ cup of blueberries

1/8 teaspoon of vanilla extract

1/8 teaspoon of ground cardamom

¼ teaspoon of ground cinnamon

5 tablespoons of divided and sliced almonds

½ cup of plain and unsweetened almond milk

½ cup of frozen sliced banana

2/3 cup of frozen raspberries

Directions

Start by placing vanilla, cardamom, and cinnamon, 3 teaspoons of almond, almond milk, banana and raspberries inside a blender. Blend the mixture until everything is smooth and well combined.

Transfer the smoothie from the blender to a medium sized bowl. Top the smoothie with the remaining 2 tablespoons of almonds, blueberries and coconut. Serve and enjoy.

26. Mediterranean Style Breakfast Couscous

Prep Time: 5 Minutes, Cook Time: 20 Minutes, Total Time: 25 Minutes

Serves 1

Ingredients

4 teaspoons of melted butter

¼ teaspoon of salt

61 teaspoons of dark brown sugar

¼ cup of dried currants

½ cup of chopped dried apricots

1 cup of uncooked whole-wheat couscous

1 (2 inch) of cinnamon stick

3 cups of low-fat milk

Directions

Start by pouring the milk in a large saucepan over medium-high heat and then add the cinnamon stick. Heat the mixture for about 3 minutes or until you start noticing small bubbles around the pot's inner edge. Ensure the mixture does not boil.

Remove the saucepan from the heat and stir in salt, currants, 4 teaspoons of brown sugar, apricots and couscous. Put a lid on the saucepan and let the mixture stand for 15 minutes. Then remove the lid from the saucepan and discard the cinnamon stick. Then divide the couscous among 4 bowls. Use 1 teaspoon of butter as well as ½ teaspoon of brown sugar as a topping for each of the bowls.

Serve and enjoy.

27. Mediterranean Oatmeal Cookies

Prep Time: 12 Minutes, Total Time: 12 Minutes

Serves 4

Calories: 380, Fat: 18g, Carbohydrates: 54g, Proteins: 9g

Ingredients

1 cup of rolled oats

½ teaspoon of salt

1 teaspoon of vanilla

2 teaspoons of cinnamon

1 cup of walnuts

1 cup of pitted dates

2 large unpeeled and coarsely chopped carrots

Directions

Start by processing the carrots until finely chopped using a food processor.

Add in salt, vanilla, cinnamon, walnuts and dates. Process the mixture for a further 30 seconds or until walnuts and dates are finely chopped. The mixture should now be able to hold together when you mold it into a ball.

Place the mixture in a large bowl and fold up the oats.

Begin to roll the mixture into 16 balls that are equal in size. Each ball should be composed of 2 tablespoons of the mixture.

Flatten the balls gently.

Serve and enjoy. You can also refrigerate the cookies in an airtight container for up to 3 days.

28. Mediterranean Pasta

Prep Time: 5 Minutes, Cook Time: 25 Minutes, Total Time: 30 Minutes

Serves 4

Calories: 360, Fat: 5g, Carbohydrates: 65g, Proteins: 13g

Ingredients

Grated parmesan cheese as topping

Pepper to taste

¼ cup of olive oil

5 cups of water

1 teaspoon of red pepper flakes

Some fresh rosemary springs

3 thinly sliced garlic cloves

1 cup of chickpeas

1/3 cup of sliced and pitted kalamata olives

2 tablespoons of tomato paste

4 cups of dried pasta

Directions

Start by placing pasta, tomato paste, kalamata olives, chickpeas, garlic, rosemary and red pepper flakes into a large skillet pan. Then lightly drizzle some olive oil on top of the ingredients and add some water.

Then cover the skillet with a lid and heat it over medium high heat until it starts to boil.

Lower the heat to low and let the mixture simmer for 15 minutes as you occasionally stir. Add pepper to taste.

Remove the skillet from the heat and discard the rosemary.

Top the pasta with grated parmesan cheese and serve while hot.

29. Mediterranean Style Breakfast Wrap

Prep Time: 10 Minutes, Cook Time: 20 Minutes, Total Time: 30 Minutes

Serves 2

Calories: 571, Fat: 22g, Carbohydrates: 80g, Proteins: 19g

Ingredients

½ cup of jarred caponata spread

1 cup of feta cheese

4 large tortillas

Salt and pepper to taste

8 eggs

2 6 ounce bags of spinach

2 cups of water

Directions

Start by heating 2 cups of water in a large nonstick skillet over medium-high heat. Then add the two spinach bags once the water starts boiling. Let the bags cook for 3 minutes or until wilted.

Remove the spinach bags and drain them by pressing them down on a colander to extort any water.

Then whisk 8 eggs, a pinch of pepper, salt and 2 tablespoons of water in a medium bowl.

Grease the earlier used skillet with 1 tablespoon of extra virgin olive oil and heat it over medium heat. Add in the egg mixture and scramble the egg for about 4 minutes or until it's just cooked.

Divide the scrambled eggs into 4 tortillas. Top all the four tortillas with 2 tablespoons of jarred caponata spread, ¼ of the spinach and ¼ cup of feta cheese. Use burrito-style to roll the tortillas.

Grease another skillet (you can as well wipe the skillet you just used) with 2 tablespoons of extra virgin olive oil and heat it over medium heat. Add in spinach wraps and cook until golden and crisp. Turn the other side and do the same.

Place the wraps on a serving plate and cut into half.

Serve while hot

30. Mediterranean Egg Casserole

Prep Time: 15 Minutes, Cook Time: 35 Minutes, Total Time: 50 Minutes

Serves 6

Calories: 308, Fat: 12.4g, Carbohydrates: 21.2g, Proteins: 27.7g

Ingredients

Salt and pepper to taste

1 teaspoon of hot paprika

¼ teaspoon of ground nutmeg

½ teaspoon of baking powder

6 eggs

¾ cup of heavy cream

1 cup of milk

6 slices of ½ inch cut fresh toast

½ cup of parmesan cheese, ground

1 ¼ cup of crumbled feta cheese

1 cup of roughly chopped fresh mint leaves with stems removed

1 cup of roughly chopped fresh parsley leaves with stems removed

1 large chopped shallot

1 large tomato chopped.

10 ounce of roughly chopped frozen artichoke (Microwave them as instructed on the package)

Directions

Start by preheating the oven to 375 degrees F. Then prepare mint leaves, parsley, chopped shallot, chopped tomato, artichokes, feta and ground parmesan and set aside.

Cut the 6 slices of fresh toast into ½ inched pieces and place them in a large bowl before setting them aside.

Take a separate bowl and whip hot paprika, nutmeg, baking powder, eggs, heavy cream, milk, salt and pepper.

Next, pour the egg mixture into the bread bowl before mixing in the cheese, the herbs and vegetables that you had prepared earlier.

Once all the ingredients are well combined, transfer them into a lightly oiled oven safe baking dish or a cast-iron skillet.

Bake the egg casserole for 35 minutes or until they are cooked through.

Slice the egg casserole into pieces and serve while hot.

Delicious Mediterranean Lunch Recipes

Below are some delicious lunch recipes that will not only make your taste buds feel like they are in heaven but will also fill you up.

31. Avocado Salad and Hummus

Prep Time: 25 Minutes, Total Time: 25 Minutes

Serves 4

Calories: 235, Fat: 12g, Carbohydrates: 26g, Proteins: 11g

Ingredients

2 ounce of shredded Gruyere cheese

1 cup of arugula leaves

½ avocado, peeled, pitted and sliced

¼ teaspoon of black pepper

4 whole-wheat split bagel bread squares or sandwich thins

1/3 cup of Mediterranean flavor hummus like Sabra Tuscan herb brand

Directions

Prepare a cooking skillet or a Panini griddle by light coating it (while unheated) with some cooking spray. Then heat over medium heat.

Next, spread the hummus on the cut surfaces of the sandwich thins. Then drizzle some black pepper, and then divide the avocado slices among the sandwich thin bottoms. Top every sandwich with avocado slices followed by ¼ cup of arugula leaves and lastly 2 tablespoons of shredded cheese.

Next, place the sandwich thin tops on the cheese and spread sides down as you lightly press down.

Place the sandwich on a skillet, griddle or a grill. If you are using a skillet, position a heavy saucepan on top of the sandwiches. However, if you are using a grill or griddle, make sure to close the lid and grill for 2-3 minutes or until the bread is nicely toasted.

Let the sandwiches cook for about 2 minutes or until the bottom part of the sandwich is toasted. Remove the lid (heavy saucepan) and turn the sandwiches over. Lid the sandwiches with the saucepan and let the sandwiches cook until the bread is toasted or for a further 2 minutes.

Serve hot and enjoy.

32. Roasted Beet and Kale Salad

Prep Time: 20 Minutes, Cook Time: 50 Minutes, Total Time: 1 Hour 10 Min

Serves 6

Calories: 129, Fat: 9.5g, Carbohydrates: 11g, Proteins: 1.7g

Ingredients

1-2 tablespoons of toasted slivered almonds

¼ thinly sliced medium red onion

Olive oil

Salt and pepper

½ teaspoon of garlic powder

½ teaspoon of dried rosemary

6 washed, dried and peeled beets

1 bunch of well washed and dried kales with ribs removed and roughly chopped

Lemon-honey vinaigrette

Salt and pepper

1 teaspoon of dried rosemary

¼ teaspoon of garlic powder

¼ cup of honey

Juice of 1 ½ lemon

¼ cup of olive oil

Directions

Ensure to prepare the ingredients as has been indicated in the ingredients section.

Then proceed to preheat an oven to 400 degrees F.

Lightly oil a baking sheet then mix a little olive oil, salt and pepper in a bowl before transferring the spinach into the baking sheet. Place the baking sheet on the oven and let them roast for about 5 minutes. Remove from the oven and set aside.

Take another baking sheet and lightly oil it. Cut the beets into 1 ½ wedges after you have peeled them. Set the beets on the baking sheet and sprinkle some pepper, salt, garlic and rosemary on them. Mix this with some olive oil ensuring to coat the beets with olive oil and spices well.

Set the beets on the oven, preferably the middle rack, and roast them for 45 minutes. Toss and turn them twice within the 45 minutes.

As you wait for the beets to roast, you can be making the lemon-honey vinaigrette. In a small bowl, combine all the vinaigrette ingredients and whisk everything to combine. Set aside.

Remove the beets from the oven and let them cool for a minute.

Use a medium sized salad bowl to combine the kale, the beets and slices of red onion. Dress the salad with the lemon vinaigrette and toss everything together.

Garnish the salad with toasted slivered almonds. Serve and enjoy.

33. Chicken Salad Greek Style

Prep Time: 20 Minutes, Total Time: 20 Minutes

Serves 4

Calories: 220, Fat: 8g, Carbohydrates: 13g, Proteins: 25g

Ingredients

Lemon wedges for garnish

¼ cup of halved pitted kalamata olives

½ cup of reduced fat feta cheese, crumbled

½ cup of thinly sliced red onion with rings separated

¾ cup of yellow sweet pepper, chopped

1 cup of halved grape tomatoes

1 ½ cups of chopped cucumber, 1 medium sized

6 cups of torn romaine lettuce

½ teaspoon of crushed dried oregano

1 teaspoon of finely shredded lemon zest

½ cup of bottled and reduced caloric Greek vinaigrette salad dressing.

2 cups of shredded chicken master recipe

Directions

Start by combining oregano, lemon zest, ¼ cup of vinaigrette and chicken in a medium sized bowl and set aside.

Toss the remaining ¼ cup of vinaigrette with lettuce in a large salad bowl. Divide the lettuce mixture among four shallow bowls by scooping 1 ½ cups of lettuce into each bowl.

Top the shallow bowls with 2 tablespoons of onion, 3 tablespoons of sweet pepper, ¼ cup of tomatoes and 1/3 cup of cucumber. Add in the chicken mixture on the center of each bowl.

Sprinkle 1 tablespoon of olives and 2 tablespoons of feta on each bowl. Serve and enjoy. If you wish, you can serve with lemon wedges.

34. Mediterranean Fattoush Salad

Prep Time: 20 Minutes, Total Time: 20 Minutes

Serves 6

Calories: 487.8, Fat: 32.1g, Carbohydrates: 32.1g. Proteins: 21.3g

Ingredients

1 cup of chopped fresh mint leaves

2 cups of chopped fresh parsley leaves with stems removed

5 thinly sliced radishes with the stems removed

5 chopped green onions

5 chopped Roma tomatoes

1 chopped English cucumber

1 heart of Romaine lettuce, chopped

Pepper and salt

½ teaspoon of sumac

Early harvest extra virgin oil

2 loaves of pita bread

Lime-vinaigrette

¼ teaspoon of scant, ground allspice

¼ teaspoon of ground cinnamon

1 teaspoon of ground sumac

Pepper

1/3 early harvest extra virgin olive oil

1 ½ lime juice

Salt and pepper to taste

Directions

Start by toasting the pita bread on your toaster oven. The bread should toast until crisp but not browned.

Oil a large pan with 3 tablespoons of olive oil and heat it up. Then break up the bread into small pieces and then place the crushed bread into the already heated oil. Toss them regularly as they fry briefly. Once they have browned, add in ½ teaspoon of sumac, salt and pepper. Remove the pita bread chips from the heat and place them on paper towels to allow them to drain before setting aside.

Make the salad. Use a large mixing bowl to combine green onions, tomatoes, cucumber and chopped lettuce with sliced parsley and radish.

Make the lime vinaigrette by whisking the spices, olive oil and lime juice together in a small bowl.

Pour in the vinaigrette mixture into the salad bowl and give it a light toss.

Add in the pita chips and sumac (optional) and toss the mixture one more time. Divide the mixture into serving plates and enjoy.

35. Quinoa Chickpea Salad

Prep Time: 10 Minutes, Total Time: 10 Minutes

Serves 1

Calories: 37, Fat: 10g, Carbohydrates: 59g, Proteins: 16g

Ingredients

A pinch of ground pepper and salt

1 tablespoon of chopped fresh parsley

1 tablespoon of unsalted sunflower seeds

½ cup of rinsed chickpeas

½ cup of cooked quinoa

2 cups of mixed salad greens

1 tablespoon of roasted red pepper, chopped

1 tablespoon of lemon juice

2 tablespoon of hummus or roasted red pepper flavor

Directions

In a small dish, stir in red pepper, lemon juice and hummus. Thin the mixture to your desired consistency with water.

Make the salad by arranging the chickpeas, quinoa and greens in a large bowl. Then top the mixture with pepper, salt, parsley and sunflower seeds.

Serve with the dressing and enjoy.

36. Griddled Chicken with Quinoa

Prep Time: 5 Minutes, Cook Time: 15 Minutes, Total Time: 20 Minutes

Serves 4

Calories: 473, Fat: 20g, Carbohydrates: 35g, Proteins: 37g

Ingredients

Zest and juice of ½ lemon

Small bunch of chopped mint leaves

100g of crumbled feta cheese

1 finely sliced red onion

Handful pitted black kalamata olives

300g of roughly chopped vine tomato

1½ tablespoons of extra-virgin olive oil

400g of chicken mini fillets

1 crushed garlic clove

1 deseeded and finely chopped red chili

25g butter

225g quinoa

Directions

Start by preparing the quinoa according to the instructions given on its pack. Rinse it in cold water and drain it thoroughly.

As you wait for the quinoa to cook, you can be making the paste by mixing garlic, chili, butter and olive oil and then set aside.

Then proceed to mix 2 tablespoons of olive oil and the seasoning before tossing the chicken fillets in. Place the chicken fillets in a hot griddle pan and let them cook for 3-4 minutes or until cooked well on each side.

Place the fillets on a plate and dot them with the earlier made paste. Set the fillets aside to melt.

Use a medium sized bowl to combine mint, feta, onion, olives and tomatoes. Toss in the earlier cooked quinoa. Next, stir in the lemon juice, the lemon zest, any remaining olive oil and then season. Top the quinoa salad with chicken fillets and drizzle with chicken juices. Enjoy.

37. Flank Steak Gyros

Prep Time: 30 Minutes, Total Time: 30 Minutes

Serves 4

Calories: 465, Fat: 18g, Carbohydrates: 45g, Proteins: 33g

Ingredients

½ cup of tzatziki sauce

4 warmed whole-wheat pitas (6-inches each)

3 cups of thinly sliced vegetables (turnips, cucumber or radishes)

1 large sliced red onion

1 cup of water

½ cup of balsamic vinegar

1 pound of trimmed flank steak

½ teaspoon of divided ground pepper

1 teaspoon of divided salt

¾ teaspoon of dried thyme

¾ teaspoon of ground cumin

¾ teaspoon of ground coriander

Directions

Start by covering a rimmed baking sheet with foil and set it aside. Position the oven rack on the upper third of the oven and then preheat the broiler to a high.

Use a small bowl to combine a mixture of ½ teaspoon of salt, ¼ teaspoon of pepper, thyme, cumin, coriander and 1 tablespoon of oil. Brush the steak with the seasoned oil and do it on both sides of the steak.

Place the steak on the baking sheet and use a small bowl to mix the onion with the remaining teaspoon of pepper and 1 tablespoon of oil. Scatter the mixture around the steak and place the baking sheet inside the oven.

Let the steak broil as you occasionally turn it. You should also stir the onions when the steak is half way through. Cook the steak for 10-15 minutes or until a thermometer registers 145 degrees F when you insert it inside the steak.

As the steak broils, mix ½ teaspoon of salt, vinegar and water in a medium sized saucepan. Heat the saucepan and let the mixture come to a boil. Add in the vegetables and cook for a further 1 minute. Remove the saucepan from the heat then slice the steak and place it on pita bread together with the tzatziki and charred onion. Drain the vegetables and add them to the steak.

Serve and enjoy.

38. Garlic Mushroom Kabobs

Prep Time: 25 Minutes, Cook Time: 20 Minutes, Total Time: 45 Minutes

Serves 6

Calories: 69.6, Fat: 4.6g, Carbohydrates: 3.1g, Proteins: 2g

Ingredients

2 tablespoon of chopped fresh parsley leaves

1 pound of cremini mushrooms

Freshly ground black pepper and kosher salt to taste

½ teaspoon of dried basil

½ teaspoon of dried oregano

3 cloves of pressed garlic

2 tablespoons of olive oil

¼ cup of balsamic vinegar

Directions

Start by preheating the oven to 425 degrees F then proceed to oil a baking sheet lightly before setting it aside.

Use a large bowl to whisk a mixture of basil, oregano, garlic, olive oil and balsamic vinegar. Season the mixture with salt and pepper to taste. Next, stir in the mushrooms and then let the mixture sit for 10-15 minutes.

Next, thread the mushrooms onto skewers then place them onto the baking sheet you prepared earlier. Then transfer the baking sheet into the oven and roast the mushrooms until they are tender i.e. for about 15-20 minutes.

Place the mushrooms on a serving plate and garnish them with parsley. Enjoy.

39. Herbed Lamb Cutlets with Roasted Vegetables

Prep Time: 15 Minutes, Cook Time: 45 Minutes, Total Time: 1 Hour

Serves 4

Calories: 429, Fat: 29g, Carbohydrates: 23g, Proteins: 19g

Ingredients

2 tablespoons of chopped mint leaves

1 tablespoon of chopped thyme leaf

8 lean lamb cutlets

1 tablespoon of olive oil

1 red onion cut into wedges

2 courgettes sliced into chunks

1 large sweet potato that is peeled and cut into chunky pieces

2 deseeded peppers (any color) that are cut into chunky pieces

Directions

Start by preheating the oven to 220 degrees C.

In a large baking tray, place the onion, courgettes, sweet potato and peppers and sprinkle over some oil. Season the mixture with a lot of ground black pepper. Place on the oven and roast for 25 minutes.

Start trimming off as much fat as you can from the lamb. Then combine the herbs with ground pepper in a small bowl and use that mixture to pat the lamb.

Remove the vegetables from the oven. Then turn the vegetables over and push them onto one side. Then place the cutlets on the already hot tray, return it to the oven and roast for about 10 minutes.

Remove the tray from the oven, turn the cutlets, and return the tray inside the oven and roast for another 10 minutes or until the lamb and vegetables are tender and lightly charred.

40. Slow Cooker Mediterranean Chicken

Prep Time: 30 Minutes, Cook Time: 6 Hours, Total Time: 6 Hour 30 Min

Serves 4

Calories: 260, Fat: 5g, Carbohydrates: 37g, Proteins: 16g

Ingredients

1 cup of long-grain white rice

1/4 cup of chopped fresh flat-leaf parsley

4 small chicken legs and 4 thighs (about 2-1/2 pounds)

1/3 cup of pitted green olives

1/2 cup of prunes

1 tablespoon of capers

6 smashed garlic cloves

3 tablespoons of red wine vinegar

Salt and pepper to taste

1-1/2 teaspoon of dried oregano

1/3 cup of white wine

Directions

In a 5-6 quart slow cooker, whisk together a combination of ¼ teaspoon of salt, vinegar, oregano, wine and pepper.

Add in some olives, prunes, capers and garlic. Give the mixture a good stir. Add in the chicken while ensuring to nestle it nicely among the prunes and olives.

Place a lid on the slow cooker and cook the chicken for 3-4 hours on high or 5-6 hours on low. Stir in the parsley.

Start cooking the rice as instructed on the package 30 minutes before serving.

Then serve the chicken with olives and prunes and the sauce over the rice. Enjoy.

41. Kale & Cannellini Stew with Farro

Prep Time: 20 Minutes, Cook Time: 3 Hours, Total Time: 3 Hours, 20 Minutes

Serves 6

Calories: 274, Fat: 4g, Carbohydrates: 46g, Proteins: 14g

Ingredients

½ cup of crumbled feta cheese (2 ounces)

3 tablespoons of fresh lemon juice

1 15 ounce can of rinsed and drained cannellini beans (white kidney beans)

4 cups of coarsely chopped fresh green kale or Swiss chard

¼ teaspoon salt

½ teaspoon of crushed red pepper

4 cloves of garlic, crushed

1 cup (2 stalks) coarsely chopped celery

Snipped fresh parsley or basil

2 thinly sliced medium carrots

1 cup of coarsely chopped onion (1 large)

1 cup of rinsed farro or kamut

1 14 ½ ounce can of fire-roasted tomatoes

4 cups of reduced-sodium vegetable broth or reduced-sodium chicken broth

Directions

Start by combining celery, garlic, carrots, onion, faro, tomatoes broth, crushed red pepper and salt in a 4-quart slow cooker.

Cover the cooker and cook the vegetables on a high-heat; cook for 2 hours or until the faro is tender but is still chewy. Next, stir in the lemon juice, beans and kales. Cover the cooker and let the mixture cook for a further 1 hour.

For serving, ensure to sprinkle each serving with parsley/basil and cheese.

42. Mediterranean Cucumber Roll ups

Prep Time: 15 Minutes, Total Time: 15 Minutes

Serves 6

Calories: 64, Fat: 5g, Carbohydrates: 3.4g, Proteins: 2.5g

Ingredients

6 tablespoons of crumbled feta

6 tablespoons of chopped roasted red pepper or sun-dried tomatoes

6 tablespoons of roasted garlic hummus

1/8 teaspoon of ground black pepper

1 large cucumber

Directions

Use a knife or a vegetable peeler to shave off thin and long slices of cucumber. One cucumber should provide you with 12 useable slices. Discard the inner slices which contain seeds.

Lay the slices down and gently sprinkle each slice with a pinch of black pepper. Spread each slice with 1½ teaspoon of hummus, 1½ teaspoon of chopped red pepper and 1½ teaspoon of crumbled feta.

Pick up one end of the cucumber slice and roll it. Do the same to all the cucumber slices. Secure the rolled cucumber slices with a toothpick.

Serve and enjoy. Ensure you don't roll them up too tightly because the filling might squeeze out.

43. Quinoa Casserole

Prep time: 15 minutes, Cook time: 45 minutes, Total time: 1 hour

Serves 4

Calories: 191, Fat: 13.4g, Carbohydrates: 12.3g, Proteins: 8.5g

Ingredients

A pinch of black pepper

½ teaspoon of salt

2 teaspoons of dried dill or ½ cup of fresh dill

6 ounces of crumbled feta cheese

½ cup of plain non-fat Greek yogurt (optional)

2 medium sized eggs

1 pint of halved cherry tomatoes

10 ounces of fresh baby spinach

2 tablespoons of olive oil

3 minced of garlic cloves

1 large yellow onion, diced

1 ½ cups of cooked brown lentils

2 ½ cups of cooked cup quinoa

Directions

Grease a large skillet with olive oil and heat it over medium heat. Add in onions and garlic. Cook for 3 minutes. Stir in the spinach and mix it with the garlic and onion. Put a lid on the skillet and let the vegetables cook for 5 minutes. Stir the mixture halfway through.

Remove the spinach from the skillet and set it on a paper towel lined plate. The paper towels are meant to absorb the excess moisture.

Preheat your oven to 375 degrees F. Oil a 9 X 13 casserole dish and set aside.

In a large bowl, mix tomatoes, spinach mixture, lentils and cooked quinoa. Set the mixture aside.

In another separate large bowl, mix dill, feta, eggs, yogurt, salt and pepper until well combined.

Add the lentils mixture to the large bowl with the feta mixture. Combine the two mixtures until everything is well coated. Transfer the mixture into the casserole dish and place it inside the oven. Let it bake for 35 -40 minutes or until the top of the casserole is golden brown.

Let the mixture cool for at least ten minutes. Serve and enjoy.

44. Spiced Salmon and Vegetables Quinoa

Prep Time: 10 Minutes, Cook Time: 20 Minutes, Total Time: 30 Minutes

Serves 4

Calories: 222, Fat: 4g, Carbohydrates: 16g, Proteins: 32g

Ingredients

Quinoa

Zest of one lemon

4 thinly sliced basil leaves

¼ cup of finely diced red onion

1 cup of cherry tomatoes, sliced into half

¾ cup of diced and seeded English cucumbers

½ teaspoon of kosher salt

1 cup of uncooked quinoa

Salmon

¼ cup of parsley

8 lemon wedges

20 ounces of salmon fillets (four 5-ounce pieces)

½ teaspoon of paprika

1 teaspoon of cumin

¼ teaspoon of black pepper

½ teaspoon of kosher salt

Directions

Use a medium saucepan to bring 2 cups of water, 1 cup of quinoa and ½ teaspoon of salt to boil. Cover the saucepan with a lid and reduce the heat to a simmer. Let the quinoa cook for about 20 minutes or until its light and fluffy. Remove the saucepan from the heat and let it sit for about 5 minutes before you serve it.

Line a sheet pan with foil and lightly coat it with olive oil or a nonstick cooking spray. In a small bowl, combine paprika, cumin, pepper and salt. Place the salmon fillets on top of the pan and coat the surface of each fillet with ½ teaspoon of the paprika mixture. The coating should be evenly distributed.

Place some lemon wedges on one side of the pan. Place the sheet pan on the lower third rack of the oven and broil on high for 8 -10 minutes or until the salmon is cooked through. You can know it is cooked when you use a fork on it and it breaks apart easily. Sprinkle the salmon with parsley.

Before serving the quinoa mixture, mix in lemon zest, basil, onions, tomatoes and cucumbers.

Serve the salmon with vegetable quinoa and roasted lemon wedges. Enjoy.

45. Italian Salad

Prep Time: 8 Minutes, Cook Time: 20 Minutes, Total Time: 28 Minutes

Serves 4-6

Calories: 480, Fat: 20g, Carbohydrates: 61g, Proteins: 19g

Ingredients

2 teaspoons of lemon zest

½ cup of toasted hazelnuts, coarsely chopped and skinned

1 peeled, seeded and diced cucumber

1 seeded and diced red bell pepper

1 cup of halved seedless red grapes

1 cup of halved seedless green grapes

2 chopped scallions

1 pound of green lentils

Vinaigrette

¼ teaspoon of freshly ground black pepper

½ teaspoon of kosher salt

1/3 cup of extra-virgin olive oil

1/3 cup of fresh lemon juice

Directions

Start by making the salad: Pour salted water in a large pot. Heat it over high heat and bring the water to a boil. Add in lentils and cook them for about 18-20 minutes or until tender. Stir regularly as the lentils cook.

Remove the pot from the heat. Drain the water and let the lentils cool for 5 minutes.

In a large salad bowl, pour the lentils and mix them with scallions, green grapes, red grapes, cucumber, red bell pepper, toasted hazelnuts and lemon zest until well combined.

Make the Vinaigrette: Pour the lemon juice in a small sized bowl. Slowly pour the oil as you constantly whisk the mixture. Make sure the mixture is well combined. Season the vinaigrette with salt and pepper to taste.

Pour the vinaigrette over the salad and toss everything together. Serve and enjoy.

46. Balsamic Lamb Chops

Prep Time: 15 Minutes, Cook Time: 8 Minutes, Total Time: 23 Minutes

Serves 4

Calories: 226, Fat: 12.1g, Carbohydrates: 2g, Proteins: 25g

Ingredients

3 tablespoons of balsamic vinegar

Cooking spray

½ teaspoon of freshly ground black pepper

1 teaspoon of kosher salt

8 (4 ounce) trimmed lamb rib chops

1 tablespoon of fresh orange juice

2 tablespoons of grated orange rind

4 teaspoons of divided olive oil

Directions

Start by marinating the lamb. Put a mixture of juice, rind and 1 tablespoon of olive oil in a large zip-top plastic bag. Add the lamb to the bag and turn it to coat. Let the lamb stand and marinate for 10 minutes in room temperature. Remove the lamb and season with some salt and pepper.

Grease a large grill pan with cooking spray and heat it over medium high heat. Place the lamb on the hot pan and let it cook for 2 minutes on each side.

Meanwhile, pour the vinegar in a small skillet that is over medium high heat. Let the vinegar cook for 3 minutes or until it is syrupy.

Place the lamb in a serving plate and sprinkle the vinegar and 1 teaspoon of oil over the lamb. Serve and enjoy.

47. Seafood with Skordalia

Prep Time: 20 Minutes, Cook Time: 35 Minutes, Total Time: 55 Minutes

Serves 4

Calories: 390, Fat: 14g, Carbohydrates: 37g, Proteins: 31 g

Ingredients

½ sliced red onion

1 pound of sliced zucchini

2 quartered red bell peppers

1 pound of halibut fillets that are cut into 4 pieces

¼ teaspoon of dried thyme

½ teaspoon of salt, divided

Zest and juice extracted from 1 lemon

3 tablespoons of divided olive oil

¼ cup of plain Greek low-fat yogurt

1 slice of sourdough bread crust removed

8 peeled garlic cloves

1 pound of Yukon gold potatoes or russet

Directions

Start by peeling the potatoes and then chop them into 1 inch pieces. Place them on a large saucepan and cover them with cold water. Add in garlic and heat the saucepan over high heat. Let the potatoes cook until they can be easily pierced with a fork. This should take about 15 minutes.

As the potatoes are cooking, rip the bread into 4 pieces and then place them on a large bowl. Then scoop 2-3 tablespoons of cooking liquid from the potatoes and then pour the liquid over the bread. Use a fork to stir the bread until the pieces are smooth. Add in 2 tablespoons of olive oil, yogurt and zest and juice of a lemon. Then stir the mixture to make a smooth paste.

Once the potatoes are ready, drain them over a large bowl that will reserve the cooking liquid for you. Add the potatoes to the bread mixture and start mashing them together. As you mash, add 2 tablespoons of cooking liquid at a time until you accomplish a loose mashed potatoes consistency. Stir in 2 teaspoons of olive oil and ½ teaspoon of salt. Cover the mixture to keep warm before you serve.

Prepare the fish. Preheat your grill pan over medium-high heat. Sprinkle the fish with ½ teaspoon of olive oil and season it with thyme and salt. Place the fish on the pan and cook it 2-3 minutes on each side or until the fish peels when you test it with a fork. Place the fish on a plate and cover it until you are ready to serve.

Prepare the vegetables. In a large bowl, combine red onion, zucchini and bell pepper. Sprinkle the remaining olive oil and toss the mixture until the vegetables are well coated. Heat the grill pan over medium heat and pour in the bell pepper mixture. Cook for 5 minutes and then add in onion and zucchini. Cook for a further 10 minutes or until the vegetables are tender. Occasionally turn as you cook.

Place the fish on one side of a serving plate, add the mashed potatoes on the other side and squeeze in the vegetables. Enjoy.

48. Bruschetta Chicken

Prep Time: 8 Minutes, Cook Time: 40 Minutes, Total Time: 48 Minutes

Serves 2

Calories: 176, Fat: 4.3g, Carbohydrates: 8.1g, Proteins: 27.6g

Ingredients

Handful of chopped basil

1/8 teaspoon of sea salt

1 teaspoon of balsamic vinegar

1 teaspoon of olive

1 clove of minced garlic

4 or 5 chopped small potatoes

3 or 4 chicken breasts

Directions

Start by preheating the oven to 375 degrees F.

Drizzle some salt and pepper over the chicken. Cover the chicken and place it on the oven. Bake it until the juices run out. This should take you 35-40 minutes.

As you wait for the chicken to bake, mix basil, sea salt, balsamic vinegar, olive oil, garlic and chopped tomatoes in a medium sized bowl. Ensure to refrigerate the salad until the chicken is ready for serving. To serve, simply place the chicken on a plate then spoon the salad over the top of the chicken.

49. Grilled Lamb Chops

Prep Time: 20 Minutes, Cook Time: 10 Minutes, Total Time: 30 Minutes

Serves 6

Calories: 238, Fat: 17g, Carbohydrates: 1g, Proteins: 20g

Ingredients

2 cloves of smashed garlic

12 small rib lamb chops

Sea salt

¼ teaspoon of red pepper flakes

½ cup of chopped packed fresh mint leaves.

1/3 cup of extra virgin olive oil

Directions

Start by preheating your grill to medium high.

In a medium sized bowl, combine red pepper flakes, mint, olive oil and salt to taste. Coat the lamb chops with garlic. Scoop a few tablespoons of the mint mixture into a small bowl and use that to brush on the chops.

Place the lamb chops on the grill and grill them for 3-4 minutes or until charred. You can test if it's ready by pressing down the middle part of the chop. If it's slightly firm then it's ready.

Transfer the lamb chops to a plate and brush them with the remaining mint oil. Then sprinkle them with some mint and serve with mint oil. Enjoy

50. Basmati Salad

Prep time: 50 minutes, Cook time: 15 minutes, Total time: 1 hr. 5 min

Serves 4

Calories: 358, Fat: 11.7g, Carbohydrates: 57g, Proteins: 10g

Ingredients

2 tablespoon of roasted pine nuts

¼ teaspoon of black pepper

1 tablespoon of olive oil

2 tablespoons of chopped fresh mint

2 tablespoons of dried currants

2/3 cup of crumbled feta cheese

½ teaspoon of salt

2 cups of hot water

1 ¼ cup of uncooked basmati rice

¼ cup of water

2 sun-dried tomatoes packed without oil

Directions

Pour the water into a small bowl and add in tomatoes. Let the tomato stand for 10 minutes. Drain the tomatoes and chop then set aside.

Put rice in a large bowl and cover it with water. The water should be 2 inches above the rice. Soak it for 30 minutes as you occasionally stir. Drain and rinse.

Mix rice and 2 cups of water into a small saucepan. Stir in the salt and heat the saucepan to medium high heat. Swirl the rice regularly as you let it boil for 5 minutes or until the water levels are below the rice. Put a lid on the saucepan, reduce the heat to a low and cook for a further 10 minutes. Remove from the heat and let it stand for 10 minutes.

Scoop the rice into a bowl and give it a light press down using a fork. Stir in feta, currants, mint, olive oil, black pepper and tomatoes. Toss the mixture until well combined. Sprinkle the rice with pine nuts. Serve and enjoy.

51. Mussels with Olives and Potatoes

Prep time: 20 minutes, Cook time: 20 minutes, Total time: 40 minutes

Serves 4

Calories: 345, Fat: 14g, Carbohydrates: 30g, Proteins: 23g

Ingredients

½ cup of roughly chopped fresh parsley

2/3 cup of halved pitted green olives

2 ¼ pounds of scrubbed mussels

1 14.5 ounce can of diced tomatoes

Kosher salt

Pinch of cayenne pepper

Pinch of allspice

½ teaspoon of paprika

4 cloves of sliced garlic

1 sliced medium sized onion

2 tablespoons of extra virgin olive oil

2 large Yukon gold potatoes cut into 1 inch chunks

Directions

Place the potatoes in a large sized microwave safe bowl. Pour in water to cover about ¼ inch. Cover the bowl with a plastic wrap and microwave it for about 6 minutes or until tender. Drain and set aside

Grease a large pot with olive oil as the potatoes cook. Then heat the pot over medium-high heat and add in onion and garlic. Cook until the onions are soft and golden brown. This should take you 5-6 minutes. Add 1 ½ teaspoons of salt, cayenne, allspice, paprika and potatoes. Stir the mixture until the potatoes have softened and are well coated with the spices. This will take 2-3 minutes.

Stir in tomatoes and a cup of water. Scrap the bottom part of the pot to remove any browned bits. Cover the large pot and let the vegetable mixture simmer for 10 minutes or until the potatoes are tender. Then proceed to stir in the olives, mussels and parsley. Cover the pot and cook for another 4-5 minutes or until the mussels open up.

Serve in a plate and enjoy.

52. Delicious Stuffed Tomatoes

Prep time: 15 minutes, Cook time: 5 minutes, Total time: 20 minutes

Serves 4

Calories: 103, Fat: 7g, Carbohydrates: 8g, Proteins: 3g

Ingredients

2 tablespoons of chopped fresh basil or thyme

2 tablespoons of Italian salad dressing or reduced fat vinaigrette

¼ cup of sliced pitted kalamata olives

¼ cup of crumbled goat cheese

½ cup of packaged garlic croutons

2 large tomatoes

Directions

Start by preheating your broiler.

Cut the two tomatoes into 4 halves crosswise. Push out the discard seeds using your fingers and cut out the pulp using a paring knife. Place the pulp on a small bowl. You should now be left with 2 tomato shells.

Lay the hollowed tomatoes on a paper towel with the cut sides down. Let them drain for 5 minutes.

Then mix basil/thyme, dressing, olives, goat cheese, croutons and pulp until well combined. Fill the hollowed tomatoes with the basil mixture.

Place the filled halved tomatoes on a broiler pan and broil 4-5 inches, away from the heat. Remove after 5 minutes or after the tomatoes are hot and the cheese have melted.

Serve while hot enjoy.

53. Eggplant with Baked Tomato

Prep Time: 15 Minutes, Cook Time: 40 Minutes, Total Time: 55 Minutes

Serves 6

Calories: 237, Fat: 6g, Carbohydrates: 42g, Proteins: 9g

Ingredients

1/4 cup of finely grated parmesan

4 tablespoons of chopped fresh basil

¼ cup of basil pesto

8 ounce of whole wheat fusilli or quinoa rotelle

1 large coarsely chopped onion

1 large coarsely chopped red bell pepper

1 halved tomato

1 eggplant cut into cubes

Directions

Heat your broiler.

Coat a large baking sheet with olive oil and arrange onions, bell pepper, tomatoes (cut side up) and eggplant on it. Coat the vegetables with olive oil. Season them with ¼ teaspoon of salt and pepper.

Place the baking sheet inside the broiler and broil for about 18 minutes or until the tomatoes are charred and the vegetables are tender and golden brown. Stir the vegetables except the tomatoes half way through cooking.

Preheat your oven to 375 degrees F. Prepare the pasta according to the package instructions. Drain the pasta and pour on a mixing bowl with 2 tablespoons of basil, pesto and the broiled vegetable. Give the mixture a slight mix and then spoon it on a baking dish. Top with cheese.

Cover the baking dish with foil and bake for 15-20 minutes. Then sprinkle the dish with 2 tablespoons of basil. Serve on a plate and enjoy.

54. Bean Salad with Zucchini

Prep Time: 15 Minutes, Cook Time: 5 Minutes, Total Time: 20 Minutes

Serves 4

Calories: 477, Fat: 28g, Carbohydrates: 43g, Proteins: 18 g

Ingredients

1 cup of crumbled goat cheese

1 cup of bulgur

¼ cup of chopped fresh dill

¼ cup of chopped roasted almonds

1 thinly sliced shallot

1 15.5 ounce can of rinsed kidney beans

2 halved and thinly sliced medium zucchini

Black pepper and kosher salt

2 tablespoon of red wine vinegar

¼ cup of olive oil

Directions

Start by making the zucchini salad. In a large bowl, mix together ¼ teaspoon of pepper, salt, vinegar and oil. Add dill, almonds, shallot, beans and zucchini. Give the vegetables a slight mix. Let the vegetables stand for 10-15 minutes as you toss them occasionally. At the end of the 15 minutes, the zucchini should be slightly soft.

Meanwhile, put the bulgur in a heatproof bowl. Add 2 cups of boiling water and cover the bowl. Let it sit for 12-15 minutes or until its tender. Drain and set aside.

Serve the bulgur on a plate and top it off with the zucchini salad. Sprinkle some goat cheese over it and enjoy the meal.

55. Root Salad

Prep Time: 25 Minutes, Cook Time: 35 Minutes, Total Time: 1 Hour

Serves 6

Calories: 197, Fat: 12.7g, Carbohydrates: 20g, Proteins: 3g

Ingredients

1/3 cup of mixed fresh herbs (parsley, dill and mint)

½ teaspoon of black pepper

1 teaspoon of salt

1/3 cup of extra virgin olive oil

2 tablespoon of whole grain Dijon mustard

1/3 cup of plain whole milk yogurt

2 tablespoons of cider vinegar

Juice of 1 lemon

2 beets with tops trimmed and cut into wedges

1 large tart apple like Granny Smith that is cut into wedges

6 radishes with tops removed

1 small celery root that is peeled and cut into wedges

2 large carrots

Directions

Process a mixture of carrots, apple, radish, beets and celery root using a food processor or a coarse grate. When processing, let the beets come in last so that it does not strain the other vegetables. Transfer the vegetables to a large bowl. Toss and set aside.

Use a separate bowl to whisk a combination of vinegar and lemon juice. Whisk in Dijon and yogurt before sprinkling in some oil. Combine the mixture until you form an emulsified dressing then season with salt and pepper.

Transfer the dressing and herbs to the root vegetables and use a spatula to toss everything together.

Serve the salad cold or at room temperature.

56. Prosciutto Toast with Avocado Cucumber Soup

Prep Time: 15 Minutes, Total Time: 15 Minutes

Serves 4

Calories: 290, Fat: 16g, Carbohydrates: 23g, Proteins: 17g

Ingredients

4 ounces of thinly sliced prosciutto

2 tablespoons of olive oil

4 slices of toasted whole wheat bread

Black pepper and kosher salt

1 teaspoon of grated lemon zest

3 tablespoons of fresh lemon juice

2 tablespoons of fresh tarragon leaves

½ cup of plain low-fat Greek yogurt

1 peeled and pitted avocado

2 peeled and chopped English cucumbers

Directions

Use a blender to puree a mixture of ¼ teaspoon of pepper, 1½ cup of water, tarragon, yogurt, avocado, cucumber, salt, zest and juice until smooth. If you desire a lighter consistency, add more water to the blender. Chill the mixture if you desire.

Lay down the toast and spread it with some olive oil. Top that with evenly divided prosciutto.

Sprinkle the soup with tarragon and serve with the prosciutto toasts.

57. Cucumber Soup

Prep Time: 20 Minutes, Total Time: 20 Minutes

Serves 4

Calories: 537, Fat: 29g, Carbohydrates: 43g, Proteins: 26g

Ingredients

½ cup of mixed olives

8 ounces of feta cheese that is broken into pieces

4 ounces of thinly sliced salami

1 small sliced baguette

Black pepper and kosher salt

3 pounds of peeled, seeded and roughly chopped cucumber

1 tablespoon of fresh lime juice

½ cup of fresh basil

2 seeded jalapenos

4 roughly chopped scallions

¾ cup of sour cream

Directions

Puree 1/4 teaspoon of pepper, ¼ cup of water, salt, half the cucumbers, lime juice, basil, jalapenos, scallions and sour cream in a blender. Add in the remaining cucumbers and puree until the mixture is smooth. Adjust the consistency of the mixture to your liking by adding water.

Serve the cucumber mixture with olives, feta cheese, salami and bread.

58. Mediterranean Cantaloupe Soup with Mint

Prep Time: 15 Minutes, Cook Time: 1 Hour 45 Min, Total Time: 2 Hours

Serves 4

Calories: 147, Fat: 0g, Carbohydrates: 37g, Proteins: 2g

Ingredients

1 ½ tablespoons of finely chopped fresh mint and small sprigs for- garnishing

½ cup of orange juice

¼ cup of honey

1 large cantaloupe

Directions

Start by halving the cantaloupe melon and hollowing out its seeds. Remove its rind and cut the fruit flesh into huge chunks. This should give you 6 cups.

Pulse a combination of honey, cantaloupe and orange juice until smooth. It can be good if you can pulse them in batches. Pour the mixture into a large bowl and cover it. Refrigerate for about 2 hours to cool.

Remove the soup from the fridge and whisk it slightly as you are sprinkling in the mint. Serve the soup in a soup bowl and garnish with springs of mint if you like. Enjoy.

59. Mozarrela Salad with Fig

Prep Time: 15 Minutes, Cook Time: 5 Minutes, Total Time: 20 Minutes

Serves 2

Calories: 286, Fat: 23g, Carbohydrates: 11g, Proteins: 10 g

Ingredients

3 tablespoons of extra virgin olive oil

1 tablespoon of fig jam or relish

3 tablespoons of balsamic vinegar

Small handful basil leaves, torn

50 grams of toasted and chopped hazelnuts

1 X 125 grams of mozzarella, drained and ripped into chunks

1 thinly sliced shallot

6 quartered small figs

200 grams of trimmed fine green beans

Directions

Place the beans in a large saucepan of water. Let them sit for 2-3 minutes before you drain and rinse them in cold water. Use a kitchen paper to drain them further.

Arrange the beans on a serving plate and top with basil, hazelnuts, mozzarella, shallots and figs.

Mix a combination of olive oil, fig jam, vinegar and some seasoning in a small bowl. Shake everything together until the liquids are well combined.

Pour the vinegar mixture over the salad and enjoy.

60. Feta Cheese Toast and Broad Bean

Prep Time: 25 Minutes, Cook Time: 4 Minutes, Total Time: 29 Minutes

Serves 2

Calories: 354, Fat: 18g, Carbohydrates: 28g, Proteins: 20g

Ingredients

4 thin slices of baguettes

1 teaspoon of lemon juice

10 halved cherry tomatoes

50 grams bag of mixed salad leaf

1 tablespoon of extra virgin olive oil

2 tablespoons of chopped and shredded mint leaves

100 grams of drained feta cheese

350 grams of fresh and frozen broad bean

Directions

In a small pan, boil water over medium heat and add beans. Let them cook for 4 minutes. Drain the beans in a colander under running water. Once the beans are cold, squeeze them out of their skin and into a bowl. Set aside.

Crush the feta cheese on a separate bowl and scatter some mint leaves over the cheese. Lightly drizzle 2 teaspoon of olive oil and season with black pepper. Toss the mixture together. Set aside

Mix the remaining olive oil with lemon juice, tomatoes and salad leaves then divide the mixture between 2 plates.

Use a toaster to toast the bread until golden and crisp on both sides.

Place the toast next to the salad. Then spoon the bean and cheese mixture onto the toasts. Serve and enjoy.

Delicious Mediterranean Dinner Recipes

This subtopic is going to highlight some of the easy to prepare dinner recipes that are not only mouthwatering but filling too.

61. Feta Shrimp

Prep Time: 5 Minutes, Cook Time: 30 Minutes, Total Time: 35 Minutes

Serves 4

Calories: 240, Fat: 8g, Carbohydrates: 16g, Proteins 25g

Ingredients

¾ cup of crumbled feta cheese

2 tablespoons of minced fresh parsley

1 pound of peeled and deveined uncooked medium shrimp

¼ cup of white wine, optional

2 cans (14-1/2 ounces each) of un drained diced tomatoes

½ teaspoon of pepper

1 teaspoon of dried oregano

3 minced garlic cloves

1 finely chopped medium onion

1 tablespoon of olive oil

¼ teaspoon salt

Directions

Grease a nonstick skillet with olive oil and heat it over medium-high heat. Add onions and cook for 4-6 minutes as you stir frequently.

Once the onions are tender, add in garlic and seasoning. Let the mixture cook for a further 1 minute.

Pour in the wine and stir in tomatoes. Let the mixture come to a boil, reduce the heat and simmer while uncovered for 5-7 minutes. The sauce should be slightly thicker by then.

Add parsley and shrimp. Continue cooking and stirring occasionally until the shrimp turns pink. This should be after 5-6 minutes.

Remove the shrimp stew from the heat and sprinkle the feta cheese. Cover the mixture and let it stand for a while or until the cheese is softened.

Serve and enjoy.

62. Pork and Orzo

Prep Time: 5 Minutes, Cook Time: 30 Minutes, Total Time: 35minutes

Serves 6

Calories: 372, Fat: 11g, Carbohydrates: 34g, Proteins: 31g

Ingredients

¾ cup of crumbled feta cheese

1 cup of halved grape tomatoes

1 (6 ounces) package of fresh baby spinach

¼ teaspoon salt

1 1/4 cups of uncooked orzo pasta

3 quarts of water

2 tablespoons of olive oil

1 teaspoon of coarsely ground pepper

1 1/2 pounds of pork tenderloin

Directions

Grease a large nonstick skillet with olive oil and heat it over medium heat.

Season the pork with pepper, and salt and then cut it into 1 inch cubes. Add the cubes to the large skillet and let them cook for 8-10 minutes or until they are no longer pink.

As the pork cooks, bring water to a boil in Dutch oven. Stir in orzo and cook for 8 minutes. Fold in the spinach and cook for a further 45-60 seconds. The spinach should be wilted after 1 minute. Drain

Add tomatoes into the skillet and let it heat for a while before you stir in the orzo mixture together with feta cheese. Remove skillet from the heat and serve.

63. Apple Beef Stew

Prep Time: 20 Minutes, Cook Time: 2 Hours, Total Time: 2 Hours 20 Minutes

Serves 8

Calories: 339, Fat: 13g, Carbohydrates: 24g, Proteins 29g

Ingredients

2 medium Fuji or gala Apples, peeled and cut into 1-1/2 inch pieces

1 tablespoon of honey

1 cup of coarsely chopped pitted dried plums

1 (14-1/2 ounces) can of beef broth

1 (15 ounces) can of tomato sauce

3 minced garlic cloves

1 large onion, chopped (about 2 cups)

2-3 tablespoons of olive oil

2-1/2 pounds of beef stew meat that is cut into 1 inch pieces

1/4 teaspoon of ground allspice

½ teaspoon of pepper

½ teaspoon of ground cinnamon

1 ¼ teaspoons salt

Hot cooked rice or couscous, optional

Directions

Start by preparing the beef. In a large bowl, mix allspice, pepper, salt and cinnamon. Sprinkle this mixture over the beef and mix to coat.

Heat 2 tablespoons of oil in a Dutch oven over medium heat. Transfer the beef into the Dutch oven and start browning the beef in batches. Add additional oil whenever necessary. Use a slotted spoon to remove the beef. Set aside.

Use the same pan to cook onions for 6-8 minutes or until they are tender. Add in garlic and cook for another 1 minute. Toss in honey, dried plums, broth and tomato sauce. Return the beef back into the pan and bring it to a boil. Reduce the heat and simmer while covered for about 1 ½ hours.

Add the apples, cover the pan and let it cook for a further 30-45 minutes or until both the apple and the beef are tender.

Serve the stew with rice. Enjoy.

64. Mediterranean Chickpeas

Prep Time: 25 Minutes, Cook Time: Total Time: 25 Minutes

Serves 4

Calories: 340, Fat: 10g, Carbohydrates: 51g, Proteins 11g

Ingredients

Dash cayenne pepper

Dash pepper

½ teaspoon of dried oregano

1 tablespoon of lemon juice

½ cup pitted Greek olives, coarsely chopped

1 (14 ounces) can of rinsed, drained and chopped water-packed artichoke hearts

1(14 ounces) can of cut up no-salt-added stewed tomatoes

1 (15 ounces) can of rinsed and drained chickpeas or garbanzo beans

2 minced garlic cloves

1 medium chopped onion

1 tablespoon of olive oil

¾ cup of uncooked whole wheat couscous

1 cup of water

Directions

Bring water to boil in a small saucepan over medium heat. Toss in couscous and remove the saucepan from the heat. Put a lid on the saucepan and let the couscous stand for about 5-10 minutes. All the water should be absorbed by then. Fluff the couscous with a fork.

As the couscous cooks, heat a large nonstick skillet with olive oil over medium-high heat. Add in onions, cook and stir until the onions are tender.

Add the garlic and cook for 1 more minute. Add in the remaining ingredients and stir until heated through.

Serve the couscous with the chickpeas. Enjoy.

65. Whole-Grain Spaghetti with Kale

Prep Time: 15 Minutes, Cook Time: 15 Minutes, Total Time: 30 Minutes

Serves 4

Calories: 413, Fat: 16g, Carbohydrates: 56g, Protein: 17g

Ingredients

¼ cup of grated pecorino, plus more for serving

1/3 cup of chopped roasted almonds

2 pints of halved grape tomatoes

1 bunch kale, thick stems removed and leaves torn into bite-size pieces

Kosher salt and black pepper to taste

2 chopped garlic cloves

1 thinly sliced medium red onion

2 tablespoons of olive oil

6 ounces of whole-grain spaghetti

Directions

Start by making pasta. Cook the pasta according to the directions given on the pasta package. Drain the pasta and save ¼ cup of the cooking water for later. Return the pasta to the pot.

As the pasta cooks, heat up a large skillet with oil over medium-high heat. Add in 1/8 teaspoon of pepper, ½ teaspoon salt, garlic and onion. Cook until the onions start to brown or for 4-5 minutes. Remember to stir regularly when cooking the onions.

Add the kale into the skillet and let the kales cook for 2-3 minutes as you frequently stir the mixture.

Add the tomatoes to the mixture and let it cook for 1 - 2 minutes. The tomatoes should be soft after 2 minutes.

Into the pot with pasta, add the reserved cooking water, pecorino, almonds and kale mixture, and mix gently

Serve and enjoy.

66. Mediterranean Grain Salad

Prep Time: 7 Minutes, Cook Time: 18 Minutes, Total Time: 25 Minutes

Serves 6

Calories: 240, Fat: 13g, Carbohydrates: 23g, Protein: 6g

Ingredients

4 ounces feta cheese, cut into small cubes

3 tablespoons of chopped fresh parsley

1 cup of pitted kalamata or black olives

1 cup of halved grape tomatoes

1-1/2 cups of cucumber slices, quartered

2 tablespoons of cold water

2 tablespoons of olive or vegetable oil

1 Box of Betty Crocker Suddenly Grain Salad Tuscan grains

Directions

Fill a 3-quart saucepan half full with water and bring to a boil. Add in the grains and bring to a boil. Boil for 17 minutes with the saucepan uncovered.

Meanwhile, make the dressing by mixing cold water, oil and dressing mix (from the salad box) and set aside.

Place the cooked grains into a colander and rinse under cold running water.

Open up the bag of grains and add in parsley, olives, tomatoes, cucumbers, packet of almonds and cheese to dressing. Mix to coat.

Serve the salad and enjoy. You can also refrigerate it and eat later.

67. Greek Burgers with Cucumber Sauce

Prep Time: 20 Minutes, Cook Time: 30 Minutes, Total Time: 50 Minutes

Serves 5

Calories: 370, Fat: 11g, Carbohydrates: 36g, Protein: 31g

Ingredients

Cucumber sauce

1 teaspoon of fresh lemon juice

2 teaspoons of chopped fresh mint leaves

½ cup of chopped cucumber

½ cup of fat-free plain yoghurt

Burgers

5 whole grain pita bread halves (6 inch)

5 thin slices medium tomato, halved

¼ teaspoon of pepper

½ teaspoon of garlic salt

1 teaspoon of crushed dried oregano leaves

¼ cup of fat-free plain yoghurt

1-1/4 lb. lean (at least 93%) ground turkey

1 (9 oz.) bag of frozen chopped spinach

Directions

Set your oven control to broil. Mix lemon juice, fresh mint, cucumber and yogurt in a medium sized bowl. Cover the bowl and refrigerate it until it's ready for use.

Follow the instructions on the spinach box to cook spinach. Let it cool drain it well.

Combine oregano, ¼ cup of yogurt, turkey, cooled spinach, garlic salt and pepper in a large bowl. Use your hands to shape the mixture into 5 oval patties with each patty being about ½ inch thick.

Set the patties on the broiler pan. Broil the patties 5 inches from the heat. This should take 10-12 minutes.

Turn the patties one time when they are halfway through. The thermometer should read 165 degree F when you insert it in the middle of the burgers.

Put 2 slices of tomato halves in pita pocket halves. Place the burgers on top of the tomato slices and top it off with 3 tablespoons of sauce. Serve and enjoy.

68. Mediterranean Pasta with Roasted Eggplant

Prep Time: 5 Minutes, Cook Time: 1 Hour, Total Time: 1 Hour 5 Min

Serves 8

Calories: 310, Fat: 5g, Carbohydrates: 53g, Protein: 12g

Ingredients

1 cup of reduced-sodium chicken broth

1 pound of uncooked multigrain pasta

Cooking spray

¼ teaspoon salt

¼ teaspoon of pepper

2 tablespoons of olive oil

1 teaspoon of dried oregano

1 onion, cut into large cubes

1 (15-oz) can of drained chickpeas

1 eggplant seeded and cut into 1 inch cubes

8 ounce container of mushrooms cut in half (optional)

6 cloves of crushed garlic

1 pint of cherry tomatoes

Granted Romano or parmesan cheese

Directions

Start by preheating your oven to 425 degrees F.

Spray a rimmed cookie sheet with the cooking spray. Add onion cubes, chickpeas, eggplant, mushrooms, garlic and tomatoes onto the cookie sheet. Add in pepper, oregano and olive oil; toss to combine.

Set the vegetables on the highest rack on the oven. Let them roast for about 55 minutes or until the vegetables have softened and turned golden. Stir the vegetables once or twice during roasting.

Meanwhile, follow the instructions on the pasta package to cook the pasta. Drain and set aside.

Remove the vegetables from the oven and pour in chicken broth.

Transfer the vegetable mixture to the cooked pasta and top with grated Parmesan cheese.

Serve immediately. If the pasta is too dry for your liking, add more chicken broth.

69. Mediterranean Kale

Prep Time: 15 Minutes, Cook Time: 10 Minutes, Total Time: 25 Minutes

Serves 6

Calories: 91, Fat: 3.2g, Carbohydrates: 14.5g, Protein: 4.6g

Ingredients

1 teaspoon of soy sauce

1 tablespoon of minced garlic

1 tablespoon of olive oil, or as needed

2 tablespoons of lemon juice

12 cups of chopped kales

Salt and ground black pepper to taste

Directions

Set a steamer insert into a pan. Fill the pan with water to a level that is just below the bottom of the steamer. Heat the pan over high heat and bring the water to a boil.

Add the kales to the steamer and steam them for about 7 10 minutes depending on the thickness of the kales. The kales should be tender after 7 or so minutes of steaming.

In a large skillet, whisk together black pepper, salt, soy sauce, garlic, olive oil and lemon juice.

Toss the steamed kales into the dressing until they are well coated. Serve and enjoy.

70. Bean Spinach Soup

Prep Time: 15 Minutes, Cook Time: 5 Hours 15 Minutes, Total Time: 5 Hours 30 Minutes

Serves 1

Calories: 148, Fat: 1g, Carbohydrates: 31g, Protein: 8g

Ingredients

8 cups coarsely chopped fresh spinach or kale leaves

¼ teaspoon ground black pepper

¼ teaspoon salt

1 teaspoon dried basil, crushed

2 cloves garlic minced

½ cup finely chopped onion

½ cup converted white rice

1 (15 ounce) can white beans, rinsed and drained

1 (15 ounce) can tomato puree

3 (14 ounce) cans vegetable broth

Finely shredded parmesan cheese

Directions

Combine tomato puree, broth, onion, rice beans, basil pepper and salt in a 4 quart slow cooker.

Cover and cook for 5-7 hours on low heat setting or for 2 ½ -3 ½ hours on high.

Stir in spinach into the soup and sprinkle some cheese. Serve.

71 Bass with Spaghetti Squash and Mushroom

Prep Time: 25 Minutes, Cook Time: 1 Hour 30 Minutes, Total Time: 1 Hour 55 Minutes

Serves 4

Calories: 432, Fat: 22g, Carbohydrates: 24g, Protein: 34g

Ingredients

4 6 ounces of striped bass fillets, pin bones removed

2 cups of cherry tomatoes

12 ounces of mixed mushrooms, cut into piece if large

Salt and freshly ground pepper

1 medium spaghetti squash

¼ cup of red wine vinegar

Pinch of red pepper flakes

1 peeled garlic head

3 or 4 sprigs of fresh rosemary

5 tablespoons of extra-virgin olive oil

Directions

Preheat your oven to 375 degrees.

Make the sauce. Add 3 tablespoons of olive oil into a small saucepan over low heat. Add in pepper flakes, whole garlic cloves and rosemary. Stir the mixture and cook for 8 minutes.

The garlic should be tender by then. Save 1 tablespoon of garlic oil. Add vinegar to the pan and let the mixture simmer over medium low heat for 5 minutes or until its syrupy and caramelized.

Halve the squash lengthwise and remove all the seeds. Brush the cut side of the squash with the garlic oil that you had reserved, and season with pepper.

Place the squash onto a baking dish cut side up and put in the oven. Let the squash roast for 1 hour or until tender.

After one hour, reduce the oven heat to 200 degrees. Remove the squash by holding it with a towel. Start pulling off its flesh in strands using a fork. Place the flesh on the baking sheet and season it with pepper. Cover with a foil and return the baking sheet to the oven to keep warm.

Heat 1 tablespoon of olive oil in a large nonstick skillet, and add in mushrooms seasoned with pepper. Cook for 10 minutes as you stir until the mushrooms are brown. Transfer the mushrooms to a plate.

Heat another 1 tablespoon of olive oil and add in tomatoes. Toss them until they blister. Add in one tablespoon of the sauce and water. Cover and cook for 5 minutes before adding in the mushrooms.

As the mushrooms cook, bring 1 inch of water to a boil in a saucepan. Season the fish with pepper and place it over the water in a collapsible steamer. Cover and steam for 5-6 minutes. Remove the fish from the heat and keep it covered for 2-4 more minutes.

To serve, place a fish fillet on a serving plate. Add in the squash, tomatoes and mushrooms. Sprinkle the food with the sauce and dig in.

72. Pancetta-wrapped Fish with Potatoes

Prep Time: 10 Minutes, Cook Time: 10-15 Minutes, Total Time: 25 Minutes

Serves 2

Calories: 521, Fat: 25g, Carbohydrates: 26g, Protein: 46g

Ingredients

4 slices of pancetta

2 tablespoons of olive oil

Zest and juice of 1 lemon

Small handful black kalamata olives

100g green bean

300g new potato

Few leaves picked tarragon sprigs

Directions

Start by heating the oven to 200 degrees C.

Add the potatoes into a pan of water over medium high heat. Boil the potatoes for 10-12 minutes or until the potatoes are tender.

Add in beans 3 minutes before the potatoes are ready. Drain the potatoes and slice them into halves. Transfer the potatoes to a baking dish, add in lemon zest, oil and olives, and toss.

Season the fish and then wrap it with pancetta. Put the fish on top of the potatoes and bake for 10-12 minutes.

Remove from the oven. Sprinkle in squeezed lemon juice and tarragon. Serve and enjoy.

73. Mediterranean Grilled Vegetable Tagine

Prep Time: 15 Minutes, Cook Time: 45 Minutes, Total Time: 1 Hour

Serves 4

Calories: 462, Fat: 7.1g, Carbohydrates: 95.5g, Proteins: 15.8g

Ingredients

¼ cup of toasted pine nuts

2/3 cup of uncooked couscous

Cooking spray

6 small red potatoes, quartered

1 (28-ounce) can of un drained diced tomatoes

¼ teaspoon freshly ground black pepper

¼ cup of golden raisins

¼ cup of sliced pitted green olives

1-1/4 cups of water, divided

¼ teaspoon of ground cinnamon

½ teaspoon of crushed fennel seeds

1 teaspoon of ground cumin

2 minced garlic cloves

1-3/4 cups of chopped onion

1 teaspoon of olive oil, divided

½ teaspoon kosher salt

2 teaspoons of balsamic vinegar

1 green bell pepper, quartered

2 red bell peppers, quartered

1 small red onion

Directions

Cut the red onion into 4 wedges and leave the root end intact.

Put the red onion, vinegar, ½ teaspoon of oil and bell peppers in a zip-top plastic bag. Seal the bag and gently toss the ingredients to coat well.

Preheat the grill. Meanwhile, in a large nonstick skillet, heat 2 tablespoons of oil over medium high heat. Add garlic and chopped onion; sauté for 3 minutes. Add cinnamon, fennel, cumin, and sauté for another 1 minute. Add potatoes, tomatoes, black pepper, raisins, olives and ¼ cup of water. Boil the mixture. Once it boils, cover the skillet, lower the heat and simmer for about 25 minutes or until the potatoes are tender.

Coat the grill rack with cooking spray. Remove the onions and bell peppers from the bag and place them on the grill rack; discard the marinade. Grill for 10 minutes as you turn the vegetables frequently.

To prepare the couscous, boil 1 cup of water in a saucepan over medium high heat. Add in the couscous and stir. Cover the saucepan and remove it from the heat. Let the couscous stand for 5 minutes, and then fluff with a fork and serve with the tomato mixture.

Top it off with red onions and grilled bell peppers. Sprinkle pine nuts over the mixture.

Serve and enjoy.

74. Cauliflower and Brussels Sprouts

Prep Time: 5 Minutes, Cook Time: 20 Minutes, Total Time: 25 Minutes

Serves 8

Calories: 72, Fat: 5g, Carbohydrates: 5g, Proteins: 2g

Ingredients

¾ teaspoon of kosher salt

½ teaspoon of freshly ground pepper

½ teaspoon of crumbled dries or 1 ½ teaspoon of chopped fresh rosemary

3 large cloves garlic, sliced as thin as possible

3 tablespoon of olive oil

2 cups (1 pint) of Brussels sprouts that is halved lengthwise

1 medium cauliflower, quartered, cored and cut into florets

Direction

Combine the Brussels sprouts and cauliflower in a large bowl. Then drizzle some oil on top and add pepper, rosemary and garlic. Mix until everything is well combined. Cover the bowl and refrigerate it overnight.

Next, preheat your oven to 450 degrees F.

Transfer the refrigerated vegetables on a large baking sheet. Spread the vegetables all over the baking sheet. Put the baking sheet on the oven and roast for 15-20 minutes or until the vegetables are crisp-tender and brown on the edges.

Serve while hot.

75. Vegetarian Pho

Prep Time: 5 Minutes, Cook Time: 1 Hour 30 Minutes, Total Time: 1 Hour 35 Minutes

Serves 4

Calories: 249, Fat: 1g, Carbohydrates: 55g, Proteins: 9g

Ingredients

4 tablespoons of prepared fried shallots, optional

1/3 cup of chopped fresh mint leaves

1/3 cup of chopped cilantro leaves

1/3 cup of chopped Thai basil leaves

2 cups of bean sprouts

2 cups of green beans, cut into 1 inch lengths

6 baby bok choy, sliced (6 cups)

7 ounces of dried rice stick noodles

2 tablespoon of Bragg liquid Aminos or low sodium soy sauce

6 cups of low-sodium vegetable broth

2 cinnamon sticks

2 tablespoons of coriander seeds

2 tablespoons of anise seeds

3 star anise

1 1-inch piece of peeled fresh ginger

1 head garlic, with the top sliced off and removed

1 medium onion, peeled and halved

Directions

Start by preheating your oven to broil. Position the oven rack at the highest position of the oven. Place ginger, garlic head and onion on the baking sheet. Put the baking sheet inside the oven and let the vegetables broil for 3-5 minutes as you turn them occasionally. Remove once they start to blacken. Place the vegetables into a large pot and set aside.

Place the cinnamon sticks, coriander seeds, anise seeds and star seeds in a small and dry skillet over medium low heat. Toast the seeds for 3 minutes or until they are fragrant.

Add the roasted spices to the onion mixture in a pot. In the same pot, add in 6 cups of water and broth. Bring the mixture to a boil and then reduce the heat to low; simmer for 1 hour with pot partially covered. Drain the broth to make about 8 cups of broth; discard solids. Put the broth back into the pot, stir in liquid Aminos, and simmer over medium low heat.

Meanwhile, cook the rice sticks according to the package instructions.

In a large pot of boiling water, cook green beans and bok choy for 4 minutes. Drain the vegetables and noodles.

Evenly divide the vegetables and noodles among 4 bowls. Pour 2 cups of broth over each bowl. Then proceed to top the beans sprout and sprinkle fried shallots as well as the herbs. Serve and enjoy.

76. Mediterranean Pressed Picnic Sandwich

Prep Time: 2 Hours 10 Minutes, Cook Time: 8 Minutes, Total Time: 2 Hours 18 Min

Serves 6

Calories: 426, Fat: 25g, Carbohydrates: 42g, Proteins: 15g

Ingredients

2 tablespoon of balsamic vinegar

1 8-ounce package of mozzarella, drained and sliced

2 jarred roasted red peppers, sliced

1/3 cup of prepared tapenade

1/3 cup of prepared pesto

1 large halved loaf of ciabatta bread

3 tablespoons of divided olive oil

1 yellow squash, cut into ¼ inch slices

1 zucchini, cut into ¼ inch slices

1 small eggplant, cut into ¼ inch slices

Directions

Start by preheating your grill pan to medium high heat.

Brush yellow squash, zucchini and eggplant with 2 tablespoons of olive oil. Grill the vegetables for 3-4 minutes and then turn and grill them for a further 3-4 minutes. They should be charred and softened. Transfer to a plate and set aside.

Cut the bread in the middle to make space for the vegetables. Apply pesto on one side of the bread and tapenade on the other side.

Lay down zucchini, eggplant, yellow squash, roasted red peppers and mozzarella on one part of the bread. Then drizzle 1 tablespoon of olive oil and balsamic vinegar before seasoning with pepper. Press the two sides of the bread together and wrap them in a tight plastic paper. Put the wrapped bread on a baking sheet and weigh it down with a large can or a heavy skillet. Refrigerate overnight or for 2 hours.

Remove from the fridge, unwrap it serve and enjoy.

1.   Spanakopita Strudels

Prep Time: 60 Minutes, Cook Time: 45 Minutes, Total Time: 1 Hour 45 Minutes

Serves 9

Calories: 223.3, Fat: 7g, Carbohydrates: 28.6g, Proteins: 11.2g

Ingredients

A cup of olive oil

1 box of thawed fillo dough (Mine sat out at room temperature for a few hours. Alternatively, you can thaw the fillo dough in the fridge overnight)

5 beaten eggs

12 ounces of feta cheese

8 ounces of cottage cheese (small curd)

10 ounces of baby spinach

Direction

Start by dividing the spinach into three batches and start placing them in a food processor 1 batch at a time. Pulse and roughly chop each batch of spinach. Place the spinach in a large bowl.

Break the cottage cheese and feta cheese into pieces and add them to the spinach bowl. Add eggs and use a spatula to stir the mixture until well combined.

Prepare the workstation that you will use to work on the fillo dough. One of the important things to have is a large cutting board and a ½ measuring cup that you will use to measure out the filling. When it comes to a measuring teaspoon, don't use the ordinary teaspoon; go for a big spoon like the one you eat a cereal with. You also need a brush which you will use to brush olive oil in the assembled strudels.

Lay down some parchment paper in a sheet pan and set aside.

Work on the fillo. Open up the fillo box, remove the fillo and place it next to the cutting board. Most fillo come in two sealed bags. So open up the first bag and unroll the fillo (fillos usually dries up very fast, so you should always roll it up gently and place it in a zip lock bag whenever you want to step away from the working station). Since you will be using a 9 X 14 inches sheet pan, you will need to cut the fillo sheet to nicely fit in your sheet pan. Prepare about 20 sheets and reserve them in a zip lock bag.

Preheat your oven to 350 degrees F. Place one sheet of fillo on the cutting board. Pour 3 tablespoons of olive oil on top of the fillo. (You do not need to brush the olive oil to coat all parts of the dough. The finished product spanakopita is actually lighter when you avoid brushing the dough with olive oil). Line another layer of fillo on top of the olive oil. Pour 3 more spoons of olive oil more specifically in the areas that were not covered on the other layer. Line one more layer of fillo and top it with 3 more teaspoons of olive oil.

Use your ½ measuring cup to dig out a level ½ cup of spinach mixture and pour it onto the fillo; about 2 inches from the bottom of the fillo. Draw the bottom part of the fillo up and over the filling. Fold sides in. Start folding the bottom part up and over itself. Keep on folding until you make a little parcel. Lay the parcel on the parchment lined baking sheet with the seam side down. Gently brush the top of the parcel with some olive oil. Repeat the whole process with the remaining fillo sheets. This will make you approximately 9-10 strudels. You probably won't be able to use up all the two bags of fillo (in this process, I used only half of the second bag of fillo).

Place the baking sheet inside the oven and bake them for 30-45 minutes or until they develop a golden brown color on top. To be on the safe side, start checking the strudels after the 30 minute mark. This will enable you to get them out before they overcook. Let them cool for a couple of minutes and then serve.

78.Mediterranean Potato Salad

Prep Time: 20 Minutes, Cook Time: 40 Minutes, Total Time: 1 Hour

Serves: 10-12

Calories: 318, Fat: 6g, Carbohydrates: 41g, Proteins: 20g

Ingredients

A large handful of fresh baby arugula leaves

A large handful of roughly chopped fresh Italian parsley leaves

1 cup of minced, pitted kalamata and green olives

¾ cup of minced red onion

3 large roasted red bell peppers with the core removed and flesh cut into strips

1 pound of fresh, tender green beans, trimmed and cut into 1 inch pieces (4 cups prepped green beans)

Salted water for cooking the potatoes

4 pounds of scrubbed clean small new potatoes or fingerling potatoes

Dressing

1/3 cup of olive oil

½ teaspoon of salt

1 teaspoon of dried tarragon (or herbes de provence)

1/3 cup of red wine vinegar

2 tablespoons of whole grain mustard

Direction

*Roast the peppers by rubbing them with some olive oil then place them on a roasting pan lined with aluminum foil under a broiler then proceed to broil until the sides become completely blackened. Turn when need be. Next, place the roasted bell peppers onto a bowl then cover it with a plate until they have cooled sufficiently. Next, carefully remove the blackened areas.

Next, place the potatoes (whole) in a large pot then pour in cold water to cover one inch above their level. Heat the pot over high heat to bring the potatoes to a simmer. Lower the heat to maintain the simmer. Cook for about 10-15 minutes or until the potatoes are able to easily pierce when you poke them with a fork. Drain potatoes and transfer them to a sheet pan to allow them to cool.

As the potatoes cook, bring another pot of water to boil and add green beans then cook for 4-5 minutes or until they are tender. Drain the beans and transfer them to an ice water bowl to immediately stop them from cooking.

Make the vinaigrette by whipping together olive oil, tarragon, vinegar and mustard in a bowl until well combined.

Then slice the potatoes into ¾ inch to 1 inch of bite-sized potatoes and place them in a large bowl. Mix with olives, red onion, bell peppers, green beans and vinaigrette. Mix together and let the vegetables marinate.

Serve the potato mixture in a plate and mix with arugula and parsley. Serve and enjoy.

79. Rustic Eggplant Moussaka

Prep Time: 1 Hour, Cook Time: 2 Hours, Total Time: 3 Hours

Serves: 6-8

Calories: 665, Fat: 49.3g, Carbohydrates: 22.6g, Proteins: 32.3g

Ingredients

Bechamel sauce

1 lightly beaten egg

¼ cup of grated parmesan, pecorino or kefalotiri cheese

1/8 teaspoon of white pepper

½ teaspoon of nutmeg

2 cups of whole milk

4 tablespoons of flour (or rice flour)

3 tablespoons of olive oil

Meat sauce

Cracked pepper

½ teaspoon of cinnamon

2 tablespoons of fresh chopped parsley

½ cup of white wine

½ teaspoon kosher salt

2 tablespoons of tomato paste

1 ½ cup of diced tomatoes (canned is ok)

1 lb. ground lamb

4 rough chopped cloves of garlic

1 large diced onion

2 tablespoons of olive oil

Eggplant

3 tablespoons of olive oil

2 lb. of eggplant

Directions

Start by preheating your oven to 400 degrees F.

Use a knife to cut the eggplant into ¼ inch pieces. Then place the eggplant on a colander and sprinkle it with salt. Stir the eggplant and let it sit for 20-60 minutes. This will make it less bitter. Rinse, pat dry and coat it with olive oil. Place it on a greased baking sheet and roast it for 20-30 minutes or until golden.

Make the meat sauce as the eggplant roasts. In a skillet heated over medium high heat, add diced onions and sauté for 3-4 minutes. Add garlic and turn heat down then sauté the mixture for another 8-10 minutes. Add in ground lamb and turn the heat to medium high. Brown the lamb for about 15 minutes as you occasionally stir. If there is any fat, drain it.

Add in pepper, cinnamon, parsley, white wine, tomato paste and diced tomatoes. Stir the mixture and cover. Turn the heat down to low and let the lamb simmer for 20 minutes.

Make the béchamel. In a large skillet over medium heat, heat 3 tablespoons of oil and whisk in 4 tablespoons of flour. Let them cook for 2-3 minutes. Whip in 1 cup of milk then mix and add another cup of milk. Stir the mixture constantly as you bring it to a boil. Reduce the heat to low and simmer for 2 minutes. Put off the heat and add in pepper, 2 tablespoons of cheese and nutmeg. Let the mixture cool. Use a separate bowl to beat an egg. Set aside.

Split the eggplant into 3 stacks. Lay down one stack of the eggplant in an 8X 13 greased pan. Top that layer with half of the meat sauce. Place another layer of eggplant and add the remaining meat sauce. Lay down the last layer of eggplant. Pour the beaten egg in the béchamel sauce and mix until smooth. Top the last eggplant layer with the béchamel sauce. Lightly sprinkle with the remaining cheese and bake it on the oven for 50-60 minutes or until it's golden at the top.

Remove from the oven. Let it cool down. Serve and enjoy.

80. Eggplant Dip (Baba Ghanouji)

Prep Time: 10 Minutes, Cook Time: 1 Hour, Total Time: 1 Hour 10 Min

Serves: 4 -8

Calories: 389, Fat: 30.76g, Carbohydrates: 26.47g, Proteins: 9.6g

Ingredients

1 tablespoon of chopped parsley

Salt and cayenne pepper to taste

Juice of one lemon- about 2 ½ tablespoons

1 teaspoon of ground cumin

1-2 finely chopped garlic cloves (use two if you like garlicky food)

2-3 tablespoons of roasted Tahini (sesame paste)

3 tablespoons of extra virgin olive oil

1-2 globe of eggplant (totaling 2 lbs.)

Directions

Start by preheating your oven to 400 degree F.

Use a fork to poke the eggplants in multiple places then slice it into half lengthwise and lightly brush the cut sides with 1 tablespoon of olive oil. Place the eggplant on a baking sheet with the cut side down. Roast the eggplant until tender. This will take you 35-40 minutes. Remove the eggplant from the oven and let it cool for 15 minutes.

Hollow out the eggplant flesh and place in a large bowl where you can mash it with a fork. Add in a pinch of cayenne, 2 tablespoons of lemon juice, cumin, tahini, olive oil and minced garlic to the eggplant. Mash the mixture until smooth. The eggplant should retain its texture.

Place the baba ghanouj mixture at room temperature to allow it to cool then season with cayenne, salt and lemon juice. You can also sprinkle it with olive oil. Top it with a sprinkle of freshly chopped parsley.

Serve with toast, celery, crackers, or cucumber slices.

81. Lentils folded into yoghurt, spinach and Basil

Prep Time: 13 Minutes, Cook Time: 7 Minutes, Total Time: 20 Minutes

Serves 4

Calories: 317, Fat: 2g, Carbohydrates: 8g, Proteins: 6g

Ingredients

Freshly ground black pepper

¼ cup of olive oil

1 cup of Greek yoghurt

1 lemon

1 finely chopped garlic clove

2 tablespoons of chopped fresh (flat- leaf) parsley leaves

1 cup of cooked lentils

1 cup of fresh basil leaves

2 cups of fresh baby spinach

½ cup of chopped pine nuts or walnuts

Directions

Use a small sauté pan over medium heat to lightly roast the walnuts or pine nuts for 5-7 minutes. Place them on a wooden cutting board to cool. Gently chop the nuts until they become almost the same size as lentils.

Tear the basil and spinach leaves into bite-sized pieces. You can also use a sharp knife that won't bruise the leaves.

Put the lentils in a large bowl and combine it with garlic, parsley, basil and spinach. Add the basil and spinach towards the end if you prefer them green. Squeeze some lemon juice into the lentils mix and then fold in the yogurt. Give the mixture another stir. Slowly pour the oil into the mixture and stir as the oil pours.

Season the mixture with pepper. Fold in the roasted nuts and top with a sprinkle of oil. Transfer the mixture to a serving plate and enjoy.

82. Greek Chicken Gyro

Prep Time: 10 Minutes, Cook Time: 15 Minutes, Total Time: 25 Minutes

Serves: 4

Calories: 195, Fat: 7g, Carbohydrates: 25g, Proteins: 10g

Ingredients

Prepare chicken gyro

4 tablespoons of crumbled feta

8 tablespoons of tzatziki

½ red onion, cut into strips

Cooked chicken

3 diced Roma tomatoes

4 pitas

Cooking the chicken

1-1.5 lbs. chicken

Pepper to taste

Zest from ½ lemon

1 clove of grated garlic, (optional)

½ tablespoon of thyme

1 tablespoon of oregano

½ lemon, juiced

1-2 tablespoons of olive oil

Directions

Start by combining pepper, lemon zest, garlic, thyme, oregano, lemon juice and olive oil in a large bowl. Mix together until well combined. Taste and adjust the seasoning. Let the mixture sit.

Add the chicken into the lemon zest marinade. Mix together to coat evenly. Cover the bowl and let the chicken marinate for 30 minutes. It works best if you refrigerate it.

Prepare your BBQ grill.

Remove the chicken from the fridge. Place on the BBQ grill and let it roast for 6-7 minutes on each side. Remove the chicken and cut it into small strips.

Make the chicken Gyro: Place the pita on the top rack of the BBQ. Let it warm for a few seconds. Remove and place on a plate.

Lay the chicken on top of the pitas. Top it with tzatziki, onions, tomatoes and feta cheese.

Serve immediately.

83. Mediterranean Salmon

Prep Time: 8 Minutes, Cook Time: 22 Minutes, Total Time: 30 Minutes

Serves 4

Calories: 339, Fat: 18g, Carbohydrates: 5g, Proteins: 37g

Ingredients

1(2 ¼-ounce) can of sliced and drained ripe olives

1 tablespoon of olive oil

2 tablespoon of undrained capers

½ cup of finely chopped zucchini

2 cups of halved cherry tomatoes

Cooking spray

4 (6-ounce) skinless salmon fillets (about 1 inch thick)

¼ teaspoon of black pepper

Directions

Start by preheating an oven to 425 degrees F.

Then proceed to sprinkle the pepper over both sides of the salmon. Grease an 11X 7 inch baking dish with cooking spray. Place the fish on the baking sheet in a single layer.

In a large bowl, mix drained olives, capers, zucchini and tomatoes until well combined. Spoon the mixture and pour on top of the fish.

Place the baking dish inside the oven and let it bake for about 22 minutes. Turn the fish when halfway through. Remove from the oven and serve while hot.

84. Crunchy Baked Mussels

Prep Time: 25 Minutes, Cook Time: 4 Minutes, Total Time: 29 Minutes

Serves 4

Calories: 301, Fat: 22g, Carbohydrates: 15g, Proteins: 11g

Ingredients

100g of garlic and parsley butter

Zest 1 lemon

50g of toasted breadcrumb

1kg of mussel in their shells

Directions

Start by scrubbing the mussels and pulling off any beards. Rinse them several times in cold water. Carefully inspect the mussels and discard any mussels that are open and don't close when tapped against a sink. Next, drain the mussels well then place them in a large pan with water. Bring the water to a boil and cover the pan. Shake the mussel mixture occasionally until the mussels open up. This will take you 2-3 minutes. Drain and discard any mussel that remained closed.

Preheat the grill to high.

Combine the zest and crumbs in a small bowl. Take out one side of the shell and lay all the shells down. Spread each mussel shell with butter and then place them on a baking tray.

Lightly sprinkle some crumbs on them and put them on the grill. Let them cook for 3-4 minutes or until crunchy.

Serve while hot.

85. Double Nut Baklava Recipe

Prep Time: 25 Minutes, Cook Time: 30 Minutes, Total Time: 55-60 Minutes

Serves 36

Calories: 174, Fat: 10g, Carbohydrates: 20g, Proteins: 2g

Ingredients

¼ cup of honey

½ cup of water

1 package of thawed phyllo dough (16 ounce, 14*9 inch sheet size)

1 ½ cup of olive oil

1 teaspoon of ground allspice

½ cup of finely chopped pecans

½ cup of finely chopped macadamia nuts

1-1/4 cups sweetened shredded coconut, toasted

Directions

Start by greasing a 13 X9 baking pan with some olive oil.

Then combine shredded coconut, a teaspoon of allspice, chopped pecans and chopped macadamia nuts in a large bowl. Mix and set aside.

Unfold the phyllo dough sheets and trim them to fit into the earlier prepared baking pan.

Arrange the 10 sheets of phyllo in the baking pan (cover the remaining doughs with a plastic wrap together with a dump cloth; that will ensure they don't dry out). Gently smear each sheet with olive oil. Sprinkle one third of the nut mixture on the sheets. Repeat the process and put 2 more layers of the nut mixture. Top with 5 phyllo sheets and brush them with olive oil.

Make diamond shapes by cutting the top phyllo sheets using a sharp knife. Bake the mixture at 350 degrees for about 30-35 minutes or until the top part turns golden brown. Place on a wire rack to cool.

Use a small saucepan to bring water and honey to a boil. Reduce the heat and let it simmer for 5 minutes. Cover the mixture and let it sit overnight.

Serve the nut baklava with honey syrup.

86. Spiced Vegan lentil soup

Prep Time: 10 Minutes, Cook Time: 45 Minutes, Total Time: 55 Minutes

Serves 4

Calories: 366, Fat: 15.5g, Carbohydrates: 47.8g, Proteins: 14.5g

Ingredients

Lemon juice made from 1 lemon to taste

1 cup of chopped fresh collard greens or kale with the tough ribs removed

Freshly ground black pepper

A pinch of red pepper flakes

2 cups of water

4 cups of vegetable broth

1 cup of lentils, picked over and rinsed

1 large can (28 ounce) of drained and diced tomatoes

½ teaspoon of dried thyme

1 teaspoon of curry powder

2 teaspoons of ground cumin

4 garlic cloves of pressed or minced

2 peeled and chopped carrots

1 medium yellow or white onion, chopped

¼ cup of extra virgin olive oil

Directions

Add one-fourth cup of olive oil to a large Dutch pot. Heat the pot over medium heat. Immediately the oil starts shimmering, add in carrots and chopped onions. Stir regularly until the onions have softened and they are translucent; this will take you about 5 minutes. Add in thyme, curry powder, cumin and garlic. Let the mixture cook for 30 seconds or until fragrant. Add in the drained tomatoes and cook for another minute or so. Stir regularly.

Pour in water, broth and lentils to the mixture. Add a pinch of red pepper flakes and season with black pepper. Raise the heat and bring the mixture to a boil. Once it has started to boil, reduce the heat and partially cover the pot. Let the mixture simmer for about 30 minutes or until the lentils are tender.

Scoop 2 cups of the lentils soup and pour it in a blender. Place a tea towel on top of the blender lid to protect your hands from the steam. Pulse the soup until smooth. Pour the pureed soup back into the lentils mixture and add in chopped greens. Let the greens cook for 5 minutes or until they are soft.

Turn the heat off and remove the pot from the cooker. Whisk in a half lemon juice. Taste the soup and season accordingly with pepper and lemon juice. Serve immediately.

87. Zucchini Mediterranean Salad

Prep Time: 20 Minutes, Total Time: 20 Minutes

Serves 2

Calories: 227, Fat: 14g, Carbohydrates: 19g, Proteins: 7g

Ingredients

2 ounces of feta cheese crumbles

8 large fresh basil leaves, torn into pieces

¾ cup of grape tomatoes, cut in half lengthwise

½ seeded yellow or orange sweet bell pepper, cut into thin strips lengthwise

1 medium zucchini, cut into ribbons (preferably with a spiralizer)

Sun dried balsamic vinaigrette

1 teaspoon of chopped sun dried tomato

1 tablespoon of aged balsamic vinegar

1 ½ tablespoons of extra-virgin olive oil

Directions

Start by making vinaigrette: Combine sun dried tomato, balsamic vinegar and extra virgin oil in a small jar. Seal the jar and shake it well. Taste the mixture and adjust the flavors to your liking.

Make the salad: Lay down zucchini ribbons between two serving plates. The ribbons should be placed in a design that will make them look like they have formed a bed for the rest of the ingredients.

Lay down the sweet pepper slices, basil leaves, grape tomatoes and feta cheese on top of the zucchini ribbons. Sprinkle the balsamic vinaigrette on the salad. Add grinds of black pepper on the salad and serve.

88. Best Roast Greek Potatoes

Prep Time: 20 Minutes, Cook Time: 60 Minutes, Total Time: 1 Hour 20 Minutes

Serves: 6

Calories: 161.8, Fat: 1.7g, Carbohydrates: 34.6g, Proteins: 3.2g

Ingredients

1 cup of parsley leaves with the stems removed

1 cup of grated parmesan cheese

1 ¼ cup of vegetable or chicken broth

Juice of 1 lemon or lime

4 tablespoons of olive oil

6 large chopped garlic cloves

Oil for baking dish

4 large baking potatoes, peeled washed and cut into wedges

1 teaspoon of rosemary or dried oregano

1 teaspoon of hot paprika

1 teaspoon of black pepper

1 teaspoon of seasoned salt

Directions

Preheat your oven to 400 degrees F.

Use a small bowl to mix all the spices and then set aside.

Wash the potatoes, peel them and then cut them into equal sized wedges. Transfer the potato wedges to a large lightly-oiled baking dish. Lightly sprinkle the spice mix over the potatoes. Toss the potatoes for them to get an even distribution of spices.

Whisk together broth, lemon juice, olive oil and chopped garlic in a medium sized bowl. Pour the mixture over the potato wedges.

Wrap the potato dish with a foil and place it in the oven. Bake for 40 minutes. Remove the dish from the oven, uncover and sprinkle parmesan cheese over the potato wedges. Place the potato wedges back to the oven; this time, they should be uncovered. Roast them for 10-15 minutes or until the potatoes have turned into a nice golden brown color.

Remove from the oven and serve while hot.

89. Swallops Provencal

Prep Time: 5 Minutes, Cook Time: 10 Minutes, Total Time: 15 Minutes

Serves 3

Calories: 349, Fat: 17g, Carbohydrates: 17g, Proteins: 28g

Ingredients

1 lemon, cut into half

1/3 cup of dry white wine

¼ cup of chopped fresh flat-leaf parsley leaves

1 minced garlic clove

½ cup of chopped shallots

4 tablespoons of olive oil

All-purpose flour, for dredging

Kosher salt and black pepper

1 pound of fresh bay or sea scallops

Directions

If you will be using sea scallops, cut them horizontally into half. However, if you are using bay scallops keep them whole. Sprinkle the scallops with pepper and toss some flour on them. Shake them off to remove any excess flour.

Heat 2 tablespoons of olive oil in a large sauté pan over high heat. Add the scallops in one layer. Lower the heat and let the scallops cook.

Once the bottom part of the scallops has lightly browned, turn it to the other side. Continue cooking until the other side browns. This will take you around 3 –4 minutes.

Pour in the remaining olive oil and add in parsley, garlic and shallots. Sauté the mixture for 2 minutes while tossing the mixture. Add wine and cook for a further 1 minute.

Taste the scallop for seasoning. If the seasoning is not enough, adjust to your liking. Squeeze some lemon juice over the scallops and serve hot.

90. Polenta and Roasted Vegetables

Prep Time: 15 Minutes, Cook Time: 50 Minutes, Total Time: 1 Hour 5 Minutes

Serves 4

Calories: 526, Fat: 27.3g, Carbohydrates: 54.9g, Protein: 15.3g

Ingredients

60g of grated cheese

4 tablespoons of extra virgin Olive oil

½ teaspoon salt

50g grated parmesan cheese

200g of fine polenta

Juice of ½ lemon

3 tablespoons of olive oil

2 red onions, cut into slim wedges

3 raw beetroot, cut into 2 cm cubes

1 butternut squash, peeled and cut into 2cm cubes

50g butter

2 teaspoons of freshly picked thyme leaf

A big handful of rocket, to serve

Directions

Preheat your oven to 200 degrees C. Cover your baking tray with a greaseproof paper or a silicone sheet.

Season the grated parmesan cheese with a pinch of black pepper, and salt. Scatter the cheese evenly on the baking tray.

Bake the cheese for 5 minutes or until golden brown. Set aside to cool. Once it has cooled, use your hands to break it into pieces.

Increase the oven heat from 200 degrees Celsius to 220 degrees Celsius. In a small baking tin, pour in a quarter cup of olive oil and lemon juice. Toss in the squash and beetroot chunks. Season with pepper, and salt and bake for 20 minutes. Remove from the oven, add in onion wedges and bake for a further 25 minutes.

As the beetroot mixture cooks, bring to a simmer one liter of water and olive oil in a large pot. Gently add in the polenta and stir regularly. Reduce the heat to low and simmer for about 35 minutes. Stir as often as possible to avoid sticking at the bottom. At this point, the polenta should be soft and thickened. Add one cup of water if the polenta starts to dry out.

Once the vegetables are ready, stir in the remaining ¼ cup of olive oil, cheese and a pinch of white pepper.

Spoon the polenta onto a serving plate. Top with any roasting juice, vegetables, rocket and thyme. Place the parmesan crisp in between the vegetables. Serve and enjoy.

Conclusion

We have come to the end of the book. Thank you for reading and congratulations for finishing my book.

I hope this book was able to help you get started on a healthy lifestyle approach to weight loss and you learned more about the Mediterranean Diet. The next step is to put what you learned into small, concrete actionable steps that will begin to change your life and help you reach your success goals!

As you have noticed, there is an endless list of foods that you can eat while on a Mediterranean Diet. The book has even done a great job of introducing you to recipes that you can prepare in the next 30 days assuming that you will be preparing a new recipe every single day!

Obviously, it would not make a lot of economic and practical sense to have a new recipe every single day. You could eat leftovers of a previous recipe, which essentially means that you can follow the guidelines in this book for more than 3 months or even for the rest of your life.

You are free to pair the recipes in whichever way you want to. If your goal is to lose weight fast, it is best to watch out how much of carb or calories you eat to ensure you don't end up taking in an excess amount of these per day, as this might mean that you have a calorie surplus that only brings about weight gain. Nonetheless, I strongly believe that the recipes in this book will still bring about effortless weight loss provided that you don't overindulge.

Now it is your turn to take action and adopt the Mediterranean Diet into your lifestyle so that it becomes a normal part of your daily routine over time.

If you found the book valuable, can you recommend it to others? One way to do that is to post a review on Amazon.

Thank you and good luck!

93115022R00128

Made in the USA
Columbia, SC
04 April 2018